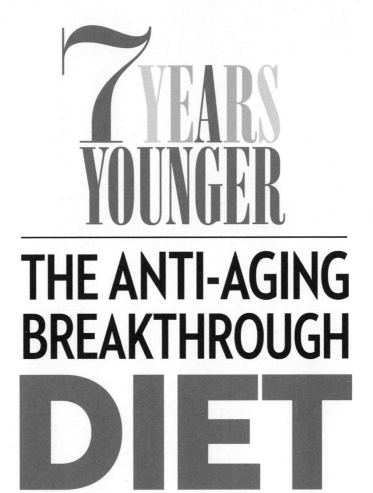

7 YEARS YOUNGER

THE ANTI-AGING
BREAKTHROUGH
DIET

7 YEARS YOUNGER

THE ANTI-AGING
BREAKTHROUGH
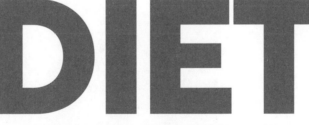
DIET

BY THE EDITORS OF
GOOD HOUSEKEEPING

An imprint of Hearst Magazines

Cont

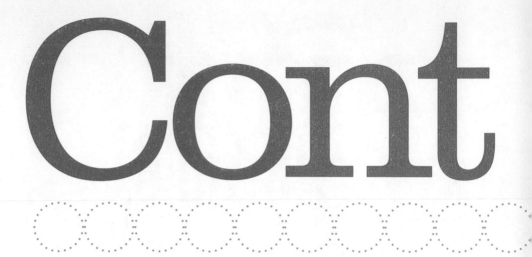

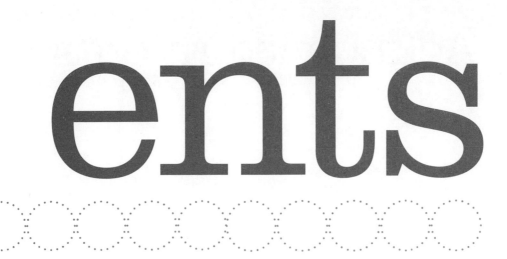

ents

Acknowledgments

I t takes a small army to produce a book this content-rich, and I am grateful to all the people who contributed their skills, insights, research, and plain old hard work. Their commitment to excellence is what propelled this project forward and created the 7 *Years Younger Anti-Aging Breakthrough Diet*.

At *Good Housekeeping*, the project was headed by Senior Executive Editor Jennifer Cook, whose expertise is surpassed only by her work ethic. Thank you, Jenny, for your editorial oversight, creative ideas, steady hand, and persistence in getting the job done right. Executive Editor Janet Siroto was also instrumental in making the book happen, organizing and working with our panelists—a gargantuan job in itself—reading and helping to edit several versions of the manuscript, and contributing her always-smart ideas.

For designing the meal plan, counseling participants, and troubleshooting food questions all the way through, my thanks go to Samantha B. Cassetty, M.S., R.D., nutrition director at the Good Housekeeping Research Institute. Also at GHRI: Susan Westmoreland and her team in the GH Test Kitchens, who developed the plan's fabulous recipes; Birnur Aral, Ph.D., Mary Clarke, and their team in the Beauty Lab; Rachel Rothman, technical manager; and Miriam Arond, director. They all deserve a week at a spa for their unstinting efforts.

Associate Editor Rachel Bowie worked tirelessly as the primary contact for our panelists on Facebook, e-mail, and beyond; Associate Editor Marnie Soman helped with research, panelist coordination, and more; and Editorial Assistants Kristin Buettner, Gabrielle Too-A-Foo, and Kathleen Corlett and Executive Assistant Shelly Watson organized the panelists' trips to *Good Housekeeping*'s offices and photo shoots. Kelly Stoddard and Heidi Cho at goodhousekeeping.com shepherded our digital efforts; copy chief Benay Bubar dotted our i's and crossed our t's. Thanks, too, to Beauty Director Nina Judar, Associate Beauty Editor Melanie Rud, Managing Editor Sarah Scrymser, and Assistant Managing Editor Dana Levy for their intelligent contributions and hard work.

Good Housekeeping Creative Director Courtney Murphy and her team in the Art Department oversaw the book's design, making sure each page was cleanly and cogently designed and doing their usual stellar work. Photo Director Bill Swan and Photo Editor Marina Harnik coordinated the panelist photo shoots and made sure they came off without a hitch. Thanks, too, to Robert Campos for laying out the book and to Jill Armus, who designed our beautiful cover.

I am also indebted to those who helped hands-on with our 7 Years Younger panelists—Michele Bender, who worked with us to find them; Nick Mastropasqua, Carissa Kelemen, and the team at Hearst Tower's The Club, who weighed, measured, and shared their expertise; and those who documented the visual results, including photographers Philip Friedman, Alex Beauchesne, and Elizabeth Griffin.

Our panelists themselves test-drove the diet and generously shared their successes, their challenges, their tips, and their criticisms, all of which proved very valuable. Thanks to each of them: Malaika Adero, Maria Arap, Debbie Barnard, Melissa Berman, Lynn Bunis, Porscha Burke, Daniel Chin, Gean Chin, Eileen Cohen, Shawna Doyle, Jeanne Fishwick, Michele Fredman, Neil Fredman, Leigh Gillam, Harvey Ginsberg, Robin Greenberg, Winston Leung, Mary Marotta, Amy Murray, Maggie Patrick, Carol Scudder, David Sigman, Arlene Ticano, Elizabeth Worthy, Jen Yamuder, and Robert Yamuder.

I'd also like to recognize the contribution of other editors from Hearst Magazines: Jill Herzig, editor in chief of *Redbook*; Sarah Gray Miller, editor in chief of *Country Living*; and Susan Spencer, editor in chief of *Woman's Day*.

Thanks to the tireless Jacqueline Deval, publisher, and TJ Mancini, product manager, of Hearst Books, and Mark Gompertz, creative director of content extensions, who coordinated with other Hearst departments on marketing and other efforts that are essential to a book's success, and to the cross-corporate SWAT team of Deede Dickson, Colleen Noonan, Laura Reid, David Schirmer, and Stephan Wasserman. Thanks, too, to Lynn Scaglione and Silvia Coppola in production, and to Christopher Dean in pre-press. And kudos to writer Deborah Yost and editor Leah Miller, whose creative efforts were instrumental in bringing this book to fruition.

This project would not exist in its multimedia form without the guidance of our marketing and digital teams. Thanks to Brian Carnahan, Tom McLean, Kim Oscarson, Sharon Bailey Romano, Elyse Lindsey, Christina Dalton, Kerry Mazzacano, Brian Madden, Ross Geisel, Charlie Swift, Liberta Abbondante, Susan Allyn, Rachel Glickman, Lauren Ruotolo, Amanda Brotherton, and Jessica Brown. Also, thanks to our video team, Scott Mebus and Valerie Volpacchio.

For creating and running the 7YY website, I thank Elizabeth Shepard, Heidi Cho, Lauren Ramakrishna, Daisy Melamed, Justin Polomcean, and Victorya Prazdnik; and for e-mail deployment and database work, thanks go to Jim Murphy, Vic Bengle, Victor Kyi, Michael Wu, and Liz Tormes.

On our 7YY newsletter team, thanks to Rose Pompeo and Ernio Hernandez, and on our social media and PR teams, to Mandi Frishman, Robin Monheit, Megan Flood, and Heidi Krupp. In accounting, thanks to Cami Pokorney, Jennifer Peltier, and Kevin Cromie, and in Marketing Creative, to Leslie Sim, Martin Danjue, Peter Wise, and Bethany Lewis.

I also want to thank my partner at GH, Senior VP/Group Chief Revenue Officer Pat Haegele—I couldn't ask for better—as well as Associate Publisher and Group Marketing Director Christine Rannazzisi Gerstein and Director of Advertising and Brand Development Sara Rad.

Finally, I want to thank David Carey, president of Hearst Magazines, for his vision and enthusiasm. Without David, neither this book nor its best-selling predecessor would have happened. Thanks, too, to John Loughlin, executive vice president and general manager, for his encouragement and support, and to other key members of the management team: Michael Clinton, president, marketing and publishing director; Ellen Levine, editorial director; Duncan Edwards, executive vice president; Debi Chirichella, senior vice president, chief financial officer; Debra Robinson, senior vice president, chief information officer; and Grant Whitmore, vice president, digital.

I hope you enjoy every page of 7 *Years Younger: The Anti-Aging Breakthrough Diet*. But more important, I hope you incorporate it into your life—and reap its rewards.

Rosemary Ellis

Editor in Chief, *Good Housekeeping*

Introduction

THE LAST DIET YOU'LL EVER NEED

Losing weight and looking younger are two dreams shared by people everywhere. Many of us—especially those of us who have labored to shed pounds only to see them creep back on again—often shrug off these goals as wishful thinking. This may be the reason you have *7 Years Younger: The Anti-Aging Breakthrough Diet* in your hands now. You want the slim figure and the burst of energy that come from terrific health, and you want to see it in the mirror, too. So, here's our promise to you: The *7 Years Younger Anti-Aging Breakthrough Diet*—developed by the same expert team at *Good Housekeeping* magazine that brought you the best-selling *7 Years Younger*—will take you there. This is the ultimate guide to shedding pounds, losing inches, and looking and feeling better than you have in years. You'll achieve your weight-loss goal and reap anti-aging benefits in just seven weeks.

It doesn't matter how many diets you've been on or how many times you've lost and gained weight. It doesn't matter how much weight you need to drop, whether 10 pounds or 110 pounds. It doesn't matter whether you're 30, 40, 50, or 60 years old, or whether you're a woman or a man.

This diet contains innovative weight-loss tools that can work for anybody. Use them—they're so easy and practical!—and you'll achieve the dream of a thinner, firmer, and more youthful body. This plan is custom-designed to make it happen, step by easy step.

A FIRST-OF-ITS-KIND APPROACH

The 7 *Years Younger Anti-Aging Breakthrough Diet* has been designed to help you permanently change your mindset about dieting, make it easy for you to adopt healthy eating habits, and provide you with a menu of irresistible foods. It's guaranteed to keep you satisfied while not overdoing it on calories. But what really makes the 7 *Years Younger Anti-Aging Breakthrough Diet* one of a kind is its emphasis on anti-aging foods. Research shows that eating the right combination of antioxidant-rich foods and following a healthy lifestyle can turn back the clock—seven full years, according to scientific reports, hence the name of this plan. The Baltimore Longitudinal Study on Aging, ongoing since 1959, has determined that the diseases often linked with getting old are not really a natural part of aging. Many of the foods that promote weight loss also fight aging. These foods protect us against heart disease, diabetes, certain forms of cancer, osteoporosis, and conditions such as mental decline. They help control blood pressure, keep good cholesterol high and bad cholesterol low, prevent insulin and blood sugar from spiking or plummeting, and fight the chronic inflammation that sows the seeds of age-related health problems. And they can return youthful luster to your skin and even help diminish wrinkles. This means your dream of losing weight, looking great, and feeling better than ever can become reality. The 7 *Years Younger Anti-Aging Breakthrough Diet* will help you turn a corner—you'll learn how to make smarter decisions about how you eat and how you move. You won't be tempted to go off this diet, because it will teach you how to make the best possible choices for your body. You'll keep the weight off because you simply won't be tempted to revert to your old habits.

Who doesn't like the idea of looking like a college kid in her 30s or being mistaken for a 30-something in her 40s? Is there anybody who wouldn't want the energy of a 20-year-old in his 50s, or who wouldn't enjoy being carded in his 70s when requesting a senior discount at the movies? Our expert nutritionists thoroughly researched the nutrients that fortify our cells against the causes of aging. Then we went in search of the foods that provide those key elements and got to work developing recipes that deliver the goods. Our nutritionists and editors worked for months putting it all together—adding here, subtracting there—to create a seven-week program featuring the healthiest and most delicious combination of vegetables, fruits, legumes, whole grains, seeds, nuts, and lean protein. These are the foundation of the 7 *Years Younger Anti-Aging Breakthrough Diet*. We've engineered these foods into a delicious, filling meal plan that delivers optimal health and weight loss in just seven weeks. The meals are both easy to prepare and designed with busy people in mind, with plenty of on-the-go options. Our plan has an ideal combination of protein, complex carbohydrates, and fat, filled to the brim with health-boosting and skin-nourishing nutrients, with a fixed amount of calories. It's all designed to produce real weight loss in a sustainable fashion, youthful energy, and health you can feel on the inside and see on the outside.

THE PROOF IS IN OUR PANEL OF SUCCESSFUL LOSERS

We know the 7 *Years Younger Anti-Aging Breakthrough Diet* works because we've put it to the test with a panel of 26 men and women, ranging in age from 34 to 62. Each had his or her own reasons for wanting to lose weight—getting back into clothes that used to fit, looking smashing for a wedding, being a better role model for the kids—but every one of them stressed a desire for better health, renewed energy, and recapturing his or her zest for life.

Over the course of the seven-week program, our weight-loss panelists stayed connected with one another and to our experts through Facebook. They were given the same food plan, the same recipes, and the same strategies for turning healthy eating into a lifestyle. Week after week, they chatted, shared tips, and encouraged one another. Each week they chatted live online with a *Good Housekeeping* expert who answered their questions. You'll see their questions and the answers throughout the book. Week 1 (our Jumpstart) went like a breeze—no hunger pangs!—with almost everybody dropping a fast few pounds. By the start of week 4, one panelist reported being down 17 pounds, while others were weighing in at 9, 13, or 15 pounds less. In all, our panelists lost a combined total of 325 pounds and 105 inches, mostly from their bellies and hips. Individual successes ranged from 3½ to 28 pounds. You'll meet many of these individuals—before and after their transformations—and read about their achievements as well as about their challenges and how they overcame them. Their queries, quandaries, and creative solutions helped us fine-tune the program to make it even easier for you.

OUR UNIQUE PROGRAM

The 7 *Years Younger Anti-Aging Breakthrough Diet* is built around our exclusive 7 Years Younger Meal Plan, engineered to turn you on to a new way of eating—one that is delicious and easy to follow. However, this is more than "just another diet." Our diet and menu plan is a strategic program aimed at turning you on to a lifestyle that's so healthy, it will turn back the clock. At *Good Housekeeping*, we believe that the best youth-restoring treatments we can give ourselves are the food we eat, the exercise we get, and the daily habits we practice. The 7 *Years Younger Anti-Aging Breakthrough Diet* is designed to deliver it all: Not only will you look better physically, but your body will actually become better equipped to resist and fight off symptoms of aging that can affect your health. It starts with taking the 7 Years Younger Diet Pledge, which you'll find on page 19. Don't skip this; it's key. As part of the pledge, you will be asked to write about your reasons for wanting to lose weight. You can keep your reasons private or share them with others, whichever you prefer. But it's critical that you make the commitment to yourself; research shows that making a formal pledge is important in helping you achieve your goal.

Chapter 1 gears you up for the diet by introducing all the wonderful benefits you'll reap from being on the plan. You'll read about the colorful bounty of delicious foods we've chosen for you and the scientific evidence that qualifies them as anti-aging foods. You'll also learn about the foods that age you, and why and how you should avoid them.

Chapter 2 offers all the enticing, mouthwatering details of the diet and the 7 Years Younger Meal Plan. We'll explore how the plan is designed to provide a simple calorie and nutrient formula you can rely on to help you lose weight *without ever feeling hungry*. All the calculations have been done for you, so all you need to do is treat this chapter like your road map for eating healthy.

There is a lot of temptation out there, but you can lick it. Chapter 3 offers creative strategies scientifically proven to help you manage cravings and keep you motivated. So, when you catch yourself with your hand in the cookie jar, you'll learn how to just brush off the crumbs and get back on track.

Experts tell us that most people who are perpetual dieters have the mindset of overeaters. It is, however, a way of thinking that science has proven can be changed. To change a habit, you've got to alter the wiring of your brain by doing things differently. In the same way it takes concentration, focus, and repetition to learn to play a musical instrument, it takes practice to rewire your circuitry from repeating bad eating habits to adopting good ones. In Chapter 4, you'll learn how to nudge your brain toward a new way of thinking about food.

Chapter 5 is about how movement and exercise can help make weight loss easier. Shedding pounds for good takes the right balance of energy (calories) in and energy out. But in addition to helping you with your weight-loss goals, getting fit also offers you the freedom to move better as you get older.

Exercise is a true turn-back-the-clock machine. While we may associate old age with diminished muscle mass, the truth is that we start losing muscle in our 30s. Lack of exercise can accelerate the risk of age-related diseases, such as heart disease and certain types of cancer. That's why in this chapter, we introduce you to four pillars of anti-aging fitness— balance, strength training, endurance, and flexibility—and show you how even the smallest changes in your routine can make a big difference in your overall health. If you aren't into exercise, we'll show you how to get inspired to start. If you do exercise but aren't feeling the benefits, we'll troubleshoot and suggest solutions. Whatever your current relationship is with exercise, Chapter 5 will help make it better.

Just tell me what to eat! If this is your approach to dieting—and it's a common one—then you'll want to dog-ear Chapter 6. It's the seven-week plan. Our team of nutritionists and dietitians, under the expert guidance of the Good Housekeeping Research Institute's nutrition director, Samantha Cassetty, M.S., R.D., carefully developed and designed the diet. Sam spent months creating this week-by-week plan, which delivers the ideal amount of nutrients, carbohydrates, fats, and protein you should eat throughout the day for maximum weight loss and optimal health and to avoid hunger. And the skin-nourishing foods she sneaked into the meals will make a noticeable difference. Just check out the before and after photos of our panelists. Your results can be similarly striking.

Eating out, whether it's fine dining or on-the-run fast food, is an American pastime, but you don't need to check your diet at the door along with your coat. Chapter 7 is all about navigating restaurant menus with ease. Yes, you can eat healthy *and* lose weight when dining away from home! We even provide a list of the best healthy options at some of America's most popular eateries to help you make choices whose taste and nutritional content you can be happy about.

Chapter 8 contains the recipes. Our panelists all gave them two thumbs up for deliciousness—one of the most important ways to judge a recipe. They are easy to make and contain ingredients you can find in any supermarket, and you should be able to prepare them in 30 minutes or less. Most of the recipes for breakfasts and lunches can be put together ahead of time or in a matter of minutes. If you need extra encouragement to try preparing your meals at home, here's some: One study found that dieters who prepare all their own food actually eat fewer calories than those who don't set foot in the kitchen.

GEAR UP FOR A CHANGE

Nobody wants to be fat, and yet today it is estimated that more than 70% of American adults are overweight. Extra poundage opens the door to killers like heart disease, diabetes, and some forms of cancer. Scientists and doctors attribute our expanding waistlines to a variety of factors—oversize portions, all-you-can-eat buffets, media messages pushing junk food, overbooked schedules that leave no time for exercise, the prevalence of computers and cell phones, television, and the decline of family recreation. There is no single cause of the rise in obesity. However, the fact remains that we simply are eating too many calories and too much of the wrong kinds of foods.

A recent multi-university study, the first to show the positive effects of calorie restriction in humans, found that the typical American diet contains 2,528 calories or more per day, with 32% coming from fat and only 16% coming from protein. When the researchers compared people who ate this way to those who ate a healthy diet consisting of a variety of nutrient-dense vegetables, fruits, nuts, eggs, fish, poultry, low-fat dairy, and whole grains—the same foods found on the 7 *Years Younger Anti-Aging Breakthrough Diet*—they found that these healthy eaters were naturally taking in more protein, less fat, and 30% fewer calories. The researchers found this group to be "significantly leaner" and significantly healthier, with hearts "comparable to [those of] healthy individuals 20 years younger."

This is not a diet with a built-in gimmick. On the contrary, it is simply a healthy way of eating that is sustainable for a lifetime. It is nutritious and contains enough calories and plenty of food to be satisfying. You'll never have to feel hungry on it. It fights aging on the cellular level, revitalizes the skin, and renews energy. And it has proven results.

Everybody has a mental vision of what they'd like to look like. When you get up each day, conjure up that vision. Tell yourself this will be the image you'll see in your mirror. Then follow the 7 *Years Younger Anti-Aging Breakthrough Diet* to make nutritious foods the focus of the way you eat; add more activity into your daily routine; and practice the strategies that will keep your diet on track and break mindless eating habits. Pretty soon, the day will come—and this is a promise—when you will say, "I've made it, and this time it's for good."

Meet The 7 Years Younger Anti-Aging Breakthrough Diet Team

⠐⠂⠐⠂⠐⠂⠐⠂⠐⠂⠐⠂⠐⠂⠐⠂⠐⠂⠐⠂⠐⠂

All Good Housekeeping projects, from magazine articles and apps to books and television shows, are collaborative. That way, we get to draw on the expertise of all our magazine editors—as well as the Good Housekeeping Research Institute directors, who evaluate more than 2,000 products annually—to bring you the most concise, up-to-date advice and information. Here's the 7 Years Younger squad:

Samantha B. Cassetty, M.S., R.D.

Nutrition Director, GHRI

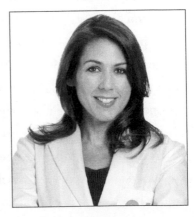

It's one thing to know which foods have the most antioxidants coupled with the fewest calories, but quite another to piece them all together into a seven-week plan. Good thing we had Sam on the job. She not only developed the weight-loss plan that anchors this book, but also was our go-to expert on all the nutrition news and facts. Sam was always on hand to help our 26 panelists figure out how to make the diet work better, choose smart substitutions, and stave off hunger. In addition to participating in Facebook chats, she was available to answer their questions; for them, it was like having a personal nutritionist (and cheerleader) on call.

Sam's nutrition and diet expertise is behind *Good Housekeeping*'s monthly *Nutrition News* and *Drop 5 lbs* columns, as well as in all of GH's weight-loss plans—including the one in our *New York Times* best-selling *7 Years Younger: The Revolutionary Anti-Aging Plan*. She has also shared her doable tips on Cooking Channel's *Drop 5 lbs with Good Housekeeping* show, now in its second season.

Susan Westmoreland
Food Director, GHRI

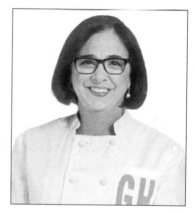

Recipes can't just *sound* healthy and delicious: To fit the 7 Years Younger standard, they must also work and be simple to make. Susan and her team in the Good Housekeeping Test Kitchens tested all of the dinner recipes that appear in this book (and our first 7 Years Younger book), tweaking them to ensure maximum flavor and minimum fuss—and every recipe passed the Triple-Test Promise, meaning that each one was tested at least three times by different cooks to guarantee that it would work in anyone's home. Susan also helps develop special issues and our extensive line of cookbooks and oversees a line of all-natural pantry products. If her name is familiar, it may be because you've seen her on television—she appears regularly on shows such as *Today* and *Good Morning America*—or you've heard her on radio shows such as NPR's *All Things Considered*.

Susan also has a video blog, *Susan to the Rescue*, and contributes regularly to the *Good Housekeeping* website.

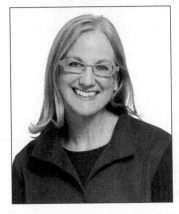

Jennifer Cook

Senior Executive Editor,
Good Housekeeping

Jenny was involved with this project from the get-go, helping to formulate the concept and then bringing it to fruition. She also helped select our panel of testers. During the writing and editing of the book, every title, every turn of phrase, and every punctuation mark was parsed by Jenny's watchful eye.

Jenny's anti-aging expertise predates 7 Years Younger and our first best-selling 7 Years Younger book. She has deep knowledge about wellness and exercise, having been a top editor at several health magazines.

Nina Judar

Beauty Director,
Good Housekeeping

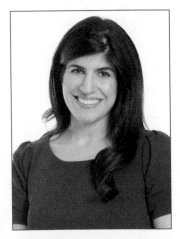

As *Good Housekeeping*'s beauty director, Nina has an expansive knowledge of skin care and hair care as well as makeup, and her electronic address book contains the names of the best dermatologists and cosmetic scientists in the business. Nina works closely with GHRI on the Anti-Aging Awards for skin, hair, and makeup, so she understands which products do the job (and which don't).

Your 7 Years Younger Diet Pledge

W riting and committing to this pledge is a vital step in the *7 Years Younger Anti-Aging Breakthrough Diet*. There's no right or wrong way to write this pledge. Yours should be personal and address exactly what matters to you. The pledge may help you find a balance between pushing yourself and setting realistic goals.

Think about the big picture: Remind yourself of all the ways in which your ultimate goal—looking and feeling younger and slimmer—will enhance your life. Also think about who will support you along the way and perhaps even include a commitment to ask for help in your pledge. Before you boot up your computer (or pull out pen and paper), take a look at the sample pledge on page 20 to give you ideas you can use when creating your own contract with yourself. (You can also see page 21 to read the pledges several of our test panelists created for their *7 Years Younger Anti-Aging Breakthrough Diet* journeys.) When you're finished, place your pledge where you'll be sure to see it every day—on your bathroom mirror, on your refrigerator door, or inside your journal.

Set aside at least 15 minutes to write your 7 Years Younger Diet Pledge. Be thoughtful, feel free to have fun and be creative, and remember to make it your own! It can be a motivating tool to remind you why you are taking this journey, especially when you slip up or feel tempted to quit. It's not set in stone; you can revise it as you go along through the upcoming seven weeks of the program and check it at the end to see how much you've accomplished. Here's an example to get you started:

7 YEARS YOUNGER DIET PLEDGE

I dedicate the next seven weeks to following the 7 *Years Younger Anti-Aging Breakthrough Diet* program.

My goal is to look and feel the very best that I possibly can.

I will invest the time and energy needed to follow the program.

I know that there will be challenging moments along the way, but with each new day I have another chance to continue the transformation that I have promised myself.

I will look to my family and friends to support me during these seven weeks and beyond, and I will support others making the same journey.

I am grateful for this opportunity to improve myself and to bring lasting positive changes into my life.

_____ Day of _____ 20 _____

_____
(Signature)

Now, as you start your diet, is a great time to get even more expert advice and ongoing support. Sign up for our free weekly e-newsletter, Your Anti-Aging Tip Sheet, *at 7yearsyounger.com/newsletter, and join us at facebook .com/7yearsyounger.*

Pledges From Our Panelists

W e asked our test panelists to think about the health, fitness, and lifestyle goals they hoped to achieve while on the 7 *Years Younger Anti-Aging Breakthrough Diet* and to write their pledges in a way that would help them focus on their goals over the course of the program. If you're having difficulty coming up with your own priorities, have a look at what they had to say for inspiration:

PLEDGE #1:

I am dedicating myself over the next seven weeks to following the 7 *Years Younger Anti-Aging Breakthrough Diet* plan, but more so, I am dedicating the rest of my life to both healthy, sensible eating habits and physical fitness. Besides the obvious goal of lowering my weight, I hope to feel better about myself and be less focused on my negative body image. In addition, I want to demonstrate the importance of healthy eating and exercise to my family and my patients (I'm a doctor). I have been a yo-yo dieter my entire life, and it is now time for it to end.

My goals for the program and afterward include fitting back into all my "thin clothes" so they no longer have to hang in my closet untouched. From a health perspective, I want to get to the point that my borderline blood sugar and prediabetic state does not progress; I hope to get off of Metformin [a diabetes drug]. My other goals include running several 5K races with my friends and ultimately participating in a half-marathon in 2014.

I know that this task will take hard work and dedication, but the time has come to take control over my health. With the support of my wife and children, I will make this happen, and I will reward myself with a new wardrobe as well as a new bicycle to ride with my friends.

PLEDGE #2:

I am fully committed to following the program and incorporating it into every aspect of my daily life. I know I will not be perfect: I will have a really bad day; I will celebrate my birthday; most likely, my father will pass away. But throughout these life events, for the next seven weeks, my commitment to the program will always be present. I am so hungry (pardon the pun) for weight-loss success, energy, confidence, and celebration that I cannot imagine losing my focus.

PLEDGE #3:

My goal is to live a healthy life by:
- *Staying spiritually connected to God*
- *Eating properly*
- *Exercising regularly*

I will succeed to the benefit of:
- *Myself*
- *My two little girls, for whom I serve as the first example of "lifestyle"*
- *My husband, who needs me to be healthy to live our lives and raise our children*

I truly realize that I look to food for comfort in stress-induced situations. I realize that stress is an everyday occurrence and I will find alternative ways to release it. These will include reading, playing with my children, exercising, researching healthy recipes, and window-shopping for clothes for the new me I envision! Also, I will establish some healthy treats as my go-to stress relievers when I just really need something.

I am excited about this opportunity and look forward to great success!

PLEDGE #4:

My goals for the Program are to start truly living my life and to stop coasting through it. The challenge I set for myself with the Program is not a transformation but a return to the confident and engaged person I remember being.

For the next seven weeks (and beyond):

- *I will be positive and not allow myself to get sidetracked by self-doubt and negativity.*
- *No more lazy food choices. I will be mindful of what I put into my body: quality over convenience.*
- *I will not be a Lone Ranger. I will reach out to my friends and family for support when I need it, and I will be supportive of my peers.*
- *I will take recess. No phone, no computer, no e-mail—a digital break for at least half an hour each day.*
- *I commit to exercising my body and mind for an hour a day. No excuses/no distractions.*

7 Years Younger Anti-Aging Resources

Take advantage of our *7 Years Younger Anti-Aging Breakthrough Diet* community!

FREE STUFF

- Get our free weekly anti-aging newsletter at 7yearsyounger.com/newsletter
- Download our free anti-aging reports, filled with helpful, doable tips:
  - *40 Best Anti-Aging Beauty Secrets* at 7yearsyounger.com/antiagingsecrets
  - *Best Anti-Aging Makeup* at 7yearsyounger.com/makeup
  - *Eat to Look and Feel Younger* at 7yearsyounger.com/eattolookyoung
  - *50 Ways to Stress Less & Live Longer* at 7yearsyounger.com/stressless

SHOPPING

- To find our top rated anti-aging beauty products, visit 7yearsyounger.com/shop
- To buy a copy of the *New York Times* best seller *7 Years Younger: The Revolutionary 7-Week Anti-Aging Plan*, go to 7yearsyounger.com/book
- To order a copy of the *7 Years Younger Anti-Aging Breakthrough Diet* Workbook, go to 7yearsyounger.com/dietworkbook
- Find out about the 7 Years Younger Plan from Nutrisystem at nutrisystem.com/7yy
- To get up-to-the-minute anti-aging, health, and diet news, subscribe to *Good Housekeeping* at 7yy.goodhousekeeping.com

SOCIAL

- Like us on facebook.com/7yearsyounger and join us there for daily tips and inspiration
- Follow us on Twitter @7yearsyounger
- Follow us on pinterest.com/7yearsyounger
- Want to be a test panelist for a future 7 Years Younger plan? Sign up at 7yearsyounger.com/panelist to be considered

Chapter 1

The Diet That Reverses Aging

D rop 10 to 25 pounds in just seven weeks. Eat foods you'll love and savor at every meal. Feel better than you have in a decade. Take years off of your appearance and melt inches from your hips, belly, and thighs.

These are big promises, we know, but the *7 Years Younger Anti-Aging Breakthrough Diet* delivers. It introduces you to a new style of healthy eating that feels so natural, you'll want to adopt it for a lifetime. It's the ultimate and essential total body makeover, designed to help you grow younger as you get thinner. It's already working for people who previously had been unsuccessful at losing weight and getting healthy, and it can work for you, too.

"The *7 Years Younger Anti-Aging Breakthrough Diet* is more than a diet; it's a lifestyle," says David Sigman, M.D., a 46-year-old physician who lost a whopping 28 pounds on the program. "I feel that I learned more about healthy eating in the first three weeks on the diet than I have in the past 45 years."

Adds panelist Porscha Burke, a book editor who lost 7 pounds: "Without sacrificing breads and cheeses and snacks, the 7 *Years Younger Anti-Aging Breakthrough Diet* shows you how to eat satisfyingly smaller portions, develop mindful eating skills, and finally institute control over your food intake—and have fun doing it."

Hundreds of studies indicate that what you eat matters more than genetics in terms of how well you age and your ability to stave off serious health problems. Anti-aging researchers say that genetics only accounts for about 25% of our risk of age-related illnesses. The rest has to do with lifestyle—most notably what we choose to eat and how active we are.

Embrace this easy-to-follow eating plan, and you can literally turn back the clock on aging. You'll feel healthier because you'll *be* healthier, with improved cholesterol, lower blood pressure, a healthier heart, more control over your blood sugar level, and a leaner body than you've had in years. One panelist said that her sleep improved, as did her menopause symptoms. And there's another surprise bonus: Studies show that these same anti-aging foods nourish your skin in a way that can help diminish wrinkles and return a glow to your skin. It's an added benefit that comes as a surprise to many, but it's a scientific fact: Eating certain foods can *improve* the texture of your skin, and on the 7 *Years Younger Anti-Aging Breakthrough Diet*, you'll be eating them every day. In fact, with its emphasis on rejuvenating nutrients, this program also helps:

- Fight obesity and target belly fat, the number one risk factor for heart disease, diabetes, stroke, and other life-threatening conditions
- Stop the chronic inflammation in the body that is believed to be at the root of many age-related diseases and health conditions
- Protect your bones and keep them strong

- Reduce "bad" LDL cholesterol and boost protective HDL cholesterol
- Normalize or reduce blood pressure
- Regulate blood sugar levels and fight insulin resistance, which can lead to type 2 diabetes
- Protect against certain forms of cancer
- Protect skin against the sun's harmful ultraviolet rays, which cause wrinkles, age skin, and increase the risk of skin cancer
- Nourish the skin and strengthen collagen, the substance that keeps it supple and discourages wrinkles, frown lines, and jowls
- Improve eye health

You will be amazed at the changes you'll experience when you follow the 7 *Years Younger Anti-Aging Breakthrough Diet*. And the first step involves recalibrating your eating habits so you will enjoy all the incredible benefits of healthy eating.

"I was honestly blown away by my results," says Winston Leung, a 40-year-old bookkeeping manager who dropped 24 pounds and reached his weight-loss goal in seven weeks. "I had no idea that it was possible to achieve such results in such a short time. I can continue eating this way for the rest of my life and not feel deprived or be afraid that the weight will come back."

THE ANTI-AGING COLOR CODE

Eating healthy may sound like a no-brainer—*More vegetables! Fewer sweets!*—but most people struggle to figure out how to eat in a way that leaves them looking and feeling their absolute best. Not only is it hard to know what to eat, but it can be equally difficult to prepare good-for-you food in a way that will be both filling and appetizing. Fifty-two

Maria Arap

"Stay positive, eat healthy, and most important, be happy!"

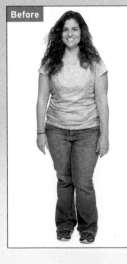

Before

Age
38

Height
5' 4"

Weight lost
10½ lbs.

Inches lost
2¼ in.

STRUGGLES IN PAST DIETING HISTORY "Different soup diets and cleanses that left me hungry and/or irritable. Starving myself or giving up stuff that I love, which didn't work. I used to snack and drink more, and now I've made an effort to limit both."

WHY 7YY "I honestly don't feel like I'm on a diet at all. 7YY is all about portion control and knowing the right stuff to eat. It is definitely a lifestyle change that I plan to stick with forever. I love the plan; it's so easy to follow!"

SUCCESS SECRET "I used to pick/sample/snack on everything. Now I make an effort not to do that anymore, because I know that 'what goes on my lips ends up on my hips.'"

PROUDEST OF "Losing weight and feeling healthy without really realizing I'm doing it."

FAVORITE 7YY RECIPES "I love all the recipes, but if I had to choose a few, I would say Turkey-Feta Burgers [page 258], Soba Noodle Bowl with Shrimp & Snow Peas [page 276], Chicken Parm Stacks [page 250], Steak & Oven Fries [page 263], and Pulled Pork on a Bun [page 260]."

BEST ADVICE FOR OTHER DIETERS "Be patient, and remember, 'Slow and steady wins the race.' The 7YY plan really works. It is a life-altering experience and a diet everyone should follow."

Want to be a panelist for a future 7 Years Younger plan? Sign up at 7yearsyounger.com/panelist to be considered.

percent of Americans say they find it a lot easier to do their income taxes than to figure out how to eat right. Well, the 7 *Years Younger Anti-Aging Breakthrough Diet* can change that. The 7 Years Younger Meal Plan that you'll find starting on page 180 tells you everything you need to know about what to eat, but we also want to give you a broader sense of what kinds of foods will serve you best. In fact, we can sum it up quite simply in one word: *color.*

The healthiest foods in the world form a colorful palette of deep, rich hues that come from antioxidants that help inhibit the inflammation and tissue damage associated with aging. These age-reversing nutrients support health in a special way. For instance, red, yellow, or orange bell peppers are a go-to anti-wrinkle food. They are brimming with vitamin C, an important wrinkle fighter because it helps strengthen collagen, a building block of healthy skin. Yellow peppers contain more vitamin C than an orange, and red peppers contain even more of it than yellow ones: Just 10 slices will give you a full day's supply of vitamin C.

In this chapter, you'll learn how various food groups can improve your health in different ways and how to best reap the benefits. In the "What You'll Eat" sections, you'll find out exactly how your meals will be balanced for the next seven weeks, beginning with the Jumpstart, so you'll get the most out of every morsel!

Mediterranean Flavor and Benefits

The 7 *Years Younger Anti-Aging Breakthrough Diet* is a Mediterranean-inspired eating plan modified for weight loss and a variety of tastes. It contains an abundance of fruits, vegetables, fish, whole grains, low-fat dairy, nuts, seeds, and olive oil—a pattern of eating that has been proven to prevent heart attack and stroke.

Fruits and Vegetables: Follow the Rainbow

The nutrients that studies show have anti-aging, disease-fighting, and skin-protecting properties number in the *thousands*, and the colorful fruits and vegetables found in the grocery store contain combinations of them all. Building your daily menu around these nutrient-dense foods will earn you a health trifecta: whittling off unwanted weight, staving off the diseases of aging, and rejuvenating your complexion.

Weight-loss stars Fruits and vegetables have long been known as "diet food" because they are low in calories. But loading up on fruits and vegetables does more than help you get thin. Israeli researchers demonstrated this when they examined how much food was consumed by people following each of three different diets to lose weight: low-fat, Mediterranean, and low-carb. The universal predictors of rapid loss of weight and the ability to keep it off two years later: an increase in fruit and vegetable consumption and a decrease in intake of sweets.

Look on the White Side, Too

White has always been associated with unhealthy, empty-calorie foods (think white bread, white sugar, etc.) But not anymore. Turning decades of nutrition advice on its head, new research has found that pale produce delivers a big health bonus. In a 10-year Dutch study of more than 20,000 people, those who ate the most white-fleshed fruits and veggies, including apples, pears, cucumbers, bananas, and cauliflower—all *7 Years Younger Anti-Aging Breakthrough Diet* foods—had a 52% lower risk of stroke than people who selected more colorful edibles.

Apples and pears were the most popular picks in the "white group," leading researchers to speculate that the benefit comes from the plant chemical quercetin in these fruits. Another major contributor of quercetin to our diet: onions. (Read about quercetin's skin benefits on page 38.)

In another study, researchers at Pennsylvania State University randomly divided 97 obese women into two groups. One group was counseled to simply reduce their fat intake, while the other was told to lower the fat in their diets and also eat more water-rich foods, particularly fruits and vegetables. After one year, all the women had lost weight, but the second group had dropped 3.3 more pounds on average (their total lost: 17 pounds).

The ultimate disease fighters Numerous studies show that the higher one's intake of antioxidant-rich fruits and vegetables, the lower one's risk of heart attack, heart disease, stroke, and certain forms of cancer. Colorectal cancer rates, for example, are highest for people who eat a high-fat diet and lowest for those who eat a nutrient-dense, high-fiber diet rich in fruits and vegetables. Eating more fruits and vegetables is also associated with a decreased risk of high blood pressure and high cholesterol and can help prevent bone loss, kidney stones, and constipation. The general rule of thumb: The deeper the color it is, the more nutrients a food contains. So pile your plate high with more fruits and vegetables to increase your protection against disease.

Super skin protectors Dozens of studies have found an association between high fruit and vegetable consumption and smoother, more resilient, better-looking skin. For example:

- A study at the University of St. Andrews in the U.K. found that people who added three portions of produce a day to their diets—no matter how much or how little of it they were eating to begin with—enjoyed a more attractive skin tone in six weeks. The volunteers rated the improvement they saw in the mirror as "even more of a beauty bonus than getting a tan," says lead author Ross Whitehead.
- A large study conducted in Italy found that people who consumed dark green leafy vegetables at least three times a week had

measurably healthier skin with less sun damage as well as a lower risk of skin cancer than people who ate the least greens.

- A British study that examined the skin of more than 4,000 women between the ages of 40 and 70 found that those with the highest intake of vitamin C-rich foods had fewer wrinkles and dewier skin.

Nutritional Skin Savers

There are certain nutrients, all part of the 7 *Years Younger Anti-Aging Breakthrough Diet*, that are so powerful, they can defend your complexion against the most skin-threatening substance on Earth—ultraviolent (UV) rays from the sun. Here they are:

- **Vitamin C,** a well-known wound healer, plays a vital role in protecting collagen. It can also help reduce dry skin. *Key sources:* bell peppers, broccoli, Brussels sprouts, oranges.
- **Vitamin D** supplies the body with the fuel it needs to replenish skin's collagen. *Key sources:* low-fat milk, yogurt, eggs, and salmon.
- **Vitamin E** has moisturizing and anti-inflammatory properties that have been shown to help diminish the effects of sun damage and inhibit the processes that cause skin aging. *Key sources:* canola oil, nuts, nut butters, and seeds.
- **Beta-carotene** increases production of collagen and glycosaminoglycans, which help your skin retain water. *Key sources:* all yellow, orange, and red fruits and vegetables.
- **Lycopene** has been found to be a strong source of sun protection and helps smooth rough skin. *Key source:* cooked tomato products (like tomato sauce).
- **Lutein** helps increase skin hydration and protect the eyes from sun damage. *Key sources:* eggs, leafy greens, broccoli,

Ask the EXPERT

Nina Judar
Beauty Director, *Good Housekeeping*

Q *I know the foods on the* 7 Years Younger Anti-Aging Breakthrough Diet *will help keep my skin looking younger. What else can I do to prevent wrinkles?*

Nina says: The sun's ultraviolet rays are a top skin ager, causing wrinkles, spots, sagging, and even cancer. To minimize sun damage, swap your plain daily moisturizer for one with sunscreen. **Follow the American Academy of Dermatology's recommendation and use a product with an SPF of 30 or higher every day.** Make sure it's labeled "broad-spectrum," meaning it follows the new FDA guidelines and protects against both UVA and UVB rays, which cause skin cancer and aging. One teaspoon will give your face protection; one ounce of a body sunscreen (a shot glass-full) will cover you from head to toe. Reapply every two hours if you are spending time outdoors. Since no sunscreen can provide 100% protection from UV damage, try to avoid being out in the sun when it's at its strongest (between 10 A.M. and 4 P.M.), and wear a hat and protective clothing. Other smart moves: not smoking, getting plenty of sleep, and eating a nutritious diet, as in the 7 Years Younger Meal Plan.

Q *With all the anti-aging lotions and potions out there, I'm confused! What should I use?*

Nina says: Even I find the drugstore aisles and department store counters confusing—there are too many choices! If you're starting from scratch, keep it simple and stick to three products: a facial cleanser, a daytime moisturizer with SPF 30, and a night cream with wrinkle fighters like retinol or peptides. These ingredients have been shown to reduce fine lines when used for eight to 12 weeks. This simple program is good for women of any age; as you get older and your skin gets drier, simply opt for a cream that feels thicker. If you want to step it up a notch, add a serum, a lightweight topical lotion with a higher concentration of anti-agers than a moisturizer. In the A.M., layer an antioxidant serum under your day cream. For the P.M., look for one with ingredients similar to those in your night cream, such as peptides.

Q *Anti-aging skin-care products are so pricey! Do I have to pay top dollar to see benefits?*

Nina says: Not necessarily. The Good Housekeeping Research Institute always tests beauty products with a wide range of prices, and our scientists have found again and again that bargain choices perform as well as—or even better than—more expensive ones. For example, the winning night cream in our first anti-aging awards, L'Oréal Paris Advanced RevitaLift Deep-Set Wrinkle Repair Night Lotion, costs about $20. However, if you're looking to spend less than that, you'll likely be disappointed. Anti-aging ingredients such as peptides and retinol tend to be more expensive than those found in plain moisturizers. One item you can always save on: facial cleanser. Dermatologists recommend Cetaphil and CeraVe, gentle face washes that are appropriate for all skin types; each costs around $10.

Q *What can I do about dark spots on my skin?*

Nina says: Start by seeing a dermatologist for a skin check, and repeat this annually: You want to be sure none of the spots are precancerous or cancerous. A skin doc can also go over speedy high-tech solutions, such as laser treatment. If you opt to fade dark patches at home with a cream or gel, patience is key: It can take eight to 12 weeks to see any improvement. The gold-standard ingredient is hydroquinone, a bleaching agent. It can be found in 2% concentration in over-the-counter skin creams, or a dermatologist can give you a prescription for a 4% concentration. Hydroquinone should be used for no more than three months and can be irritating. Retinoic acid, a vitamin A derivative, can minimize spots and wrinkles simultaneously, especially when used at prescription strength. Most skin tone-evening creams sold in stores contain retinol—a less potent vitamin A derivative—or a host of other ingredients such as vitamin C and licorice extract. Though these are generally not irritating, they're also not as effective as retinoic acid. No matter what you use, minimize sun exposure and wear SPF 30 sunscreen daily—otherwise, the spots will return.

Find top rated anti-aging products at 7yearsyounger.com/shop.

corn, and peas.

- **Selenium** offers protection against the sun. *Key sources:* eggs, mushrooms, whole grains, salmon, tuna, lean pork, and poultry.
- **Zinc** helps break down damaged collagen, clearing the way for renewal of elasticity and smoothing surface lines in the skin. *Key sources:* lean meats, shellfish, and beans.
- Other well-known skin protectors include **flavonoids**, found in red grapes, blueberries, strawberries, and red cabbage; **quercetin,** found in onions, apples, berries, and broccoli; **isoflavones,** found in soybeans; and **ellagic acid,** found in berries and pomegranates.

What you'll eat The wider the variety of colorful fruits and vegetables you eat, the more benefits you'll reap. The 7 *Years Younger Anti-Aging Breakthrough Diet* fills at least half of your plate with fruits and vegetables

Snack Your Way to Smoother Skin

BONUS TIP

A multinational study involving 453 people living in Australia, Greece, Japan, and Sweden found a link between the quality of a person's diet and his or her number of facial wrinkles. Fewer wrinkles were associated with the highest intake of vegetables, legumes, and olive oil—all *7 Years Younger Anti-Aging Breakthrough Diet* foods. The most wrinkling was associated with the diets highest in sugar, whole milk, butter, margarine, and red meat. On the *7 Years Younger Anti-Aging Breakthrough Diet*, you'll learn how to reduce your intake of those foods in ways that are so delicious, you won't even miss them.

at every meal.

"The best thing about this plan is the strategic nature of the eating," says Carol Scudder-Danilowicz, a 51-year-old caterer who lost 8½ pounds. "It's the gift that keeps on giving. People want to know what I'm doing. They're asking for recipes and want tips. It's great to finally be on a program that works—and one that isn't about sacrifice."

Protein: Essential at Every Meal

Easier weight loss We start losing muscle in our 30s, and by age 40, muscle mass, or what doctors call lean body tissue, begins to decline by up to 1% a year. This drop in lean body tissue slows metabolism, which allows pounds to creep on. It's the primary reason that weight loss gets tougher as we get older.

Eating more protein, however, will make it easier to lose weight; the calories from protein do a much better job at filling you up and keeping you full than just about anything else you eat. That means you're more likely to be satisfied with less food, so the pounds will come off without hunger pangs. Plus, protein gives your body the nutrients to build and replace lean body tissue. In fact, we've built more of it into the 7 *Years Younger Anti-Aging Breakthrough Diet* than even the USDA recommends. It is an essential muscle booster and skin saver; that's the reason you'll find protein in every one of our meals. Since muscle is metabolically active,

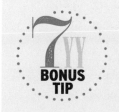

Slash the Fat

Here's an effortless and easy way to trim fat from your meals: Swap out red meat for poultry, fish, or legumes. Each time you do, you'll cut your intake of saturated fat by 15%.

Be Calorie-Conscious in Choosing Meats

You'll find plenty of meat in our meal plan, all of it quality cuts–beef and pork tenderloin and skinless chicken breasts, for example. As you'll see in this swap list, the cut really does make a big fat difference. Some of these choices might cost you a little more money, but you'll save big on calories when you choose the leanest cuts of meat and poultry–not to mention what you'll save on health care costs down the road. Think of it as an investment in your future!

Swap...	for...	and save...
Pork ribs 558 cals	Pork tenderloin 250 cals	308 cals
Prime rib 480 cals	Beef tenderloin 240 cals	240 cals
70% lean ground beef 464 cals	95% lean ground beef 291 cals	173 cals
Chicken leg with skin 394 cals	Skinless chicken breast 289 cals	105 cals

having more of it means you'll burn calories more efficiently. The more muscle you build—and, yes, the 7 *Years Younger Anti-Aging Breakthrough Diet* fits exercise into the formula—the higher your metabolism will be.

A prime muscle builder Excess weight means excess fat that puts your health at risk. Down the road, diminished muscle mass can throw your equilibrium off balance—upping your chances of a fall, sapping your energy, and even threatening your ability to recover from an accident or illness.

As part of the Framingham Osteoporosis Study, researchers looked at the protein intake of more than 900 men and women with an average age of 75. They found that those who ate the most protein had a significantly lower risk of hip fracture. Since bone density didn't differ much among them, the researchers believe eating protein might have helped prevent breaks by increasing muscle mass and strength in their lower bodies.

Wrinkle eraser People who eat the most protein have the smoothest skin, according to the results of a British study. Protein provides the building blocks of collagen, says F. William Danby, M.D., adjunct professor of surgery (dermatology) at Dartmouth Medical School. Collagen is critical to how plump and healthy your skin looks.

Your skin will make collagen whether you dine on marbled steaks or skinless chicken breasts, but the leaner choice will help you lose weight. Red meats, which are high in saturated fat, are thought to contribute to heart disease and certain forms of cancer.

What you'll eat A key to making sure every meal leaves you feeling full and satisfied is getting enough protein. And there are plenty of options: beans, low-fat dairy, eggs, legumes, seafood, and lean cuts of meat and poultry. A nonmeat source of protein you'll find on the 7 *Years Younger Anti-Aging Breakthrough Diet* is tofu, a whole soy food. Though the research isn't definitive, a small Japanese study found that women who consumed soy extract for 12 weeks had greater elasticity in their skin and fewer fine lines around their eyes than women who got less soy in their diets.

Dairy: The Low-Fat Way to Go

Dairy is an excellent source of calcium and vitamin D and can be an important protein source—one cup of milk offers 8 grams of protein, more than you get from eating an egg. It is also rich in minerals and nutrients that are tied to positive health benefits. Yet many experts believe that about two-thirds of Americans don't get enough dairy in their diets.

Calcium Dairy foods are packed with calcium, the nutrient important to

Wean Yourself Off Whole Milk

Even if you grew up loving whole milk, you can train your taste buds to get just as much enjoyment out of a lower-fat version. Just cut back gradually. After a while, you'll likely find that whole milk tastes too rich.

Ideally, your goal should be 1% or fat-free. Whole milk, for example, contains roughly 3.25% milk fat, so dropping to 2% milk doesn't offer much of a reduction: It's better than whole milk, but it still has 5 grams of fat, 3 of which are the artery-clogging saturated variety. If you shy away from skim milk, the best choice is 1%, at 2.5 grams of fat with 1.5 of those grams being saturated.

Your best bet may be the protein-fortified "plus" fat-free milk. It tastes creamier than regular fat-free.

strong bones. Bone loss begins in your 30s, and in women, it accelerates after menopause as levels of estrogen diminish. Weight-bearing physical activity, such as walking, is critical for saving bone mass, but diet is important, too—that's why we should embrace dairy foods. (Bone health also gets a big assist from the protein found in dairy.)

Vitamin D One reason the 7 *Years Younger Anti-Aging Breakthrough Diet* is filled with dairy foods is that they are fortified with vitamin D, a nutrient getting a lot of attention these days as an important safeguard against age-related disease and a help in delaying the aging process.

Other notable nutrients Foods like milk, yogurt, and cheese are key sources of potassium, phosphorus, riboflavin, and niacin, and they're packed into our meal plan because they're associated with numerous benefits, such as keeping your cardiovascular system young and vital, reducing blood pressure, and lowering the risk of type 2 diabetes and colon cancer. Studies show that dieters may also get an added weight-loss edge by including dairy on their daily menu.

The evidence for dairy foods' benefits keeps mounting. A Japanese study found that eating just a quarter-cup of yogurt a day led to a 50% reduction in tooth loss and a 60% lower risk of heart disease, most likely attributable to the beneficial bacteria known as probiotics found in yogurt (look for "live, active cultures" on the label). Probiotics are also linked with additional health perks such as improved immunity and digestion.

One thing to keep in mind: The fat in dairy does nothing to supply you with health-sustaining nutrients, which is why we recommend using mainly low-fat dairy products.

Fish: Eat It to Your Heart's Content

Health experts are pleading for people to eat more fish because it is the richest source of omega-3 fatty acids and the *only* direct source of the most important two: eicosapentaenoic acid (EPA) and docosahexaenoic acid (DHA).

Although most seafood has some healthy fats, the kinds of fish that offer you the most benefits are oily varieties such as salmon, tuna, halibut, and trout. Even fish get cold swimming in frigid water, and these species build up layers of fatty tissue that act as insulation. It turns out that fish oil from that fat offers special protection to humans as well, mostly notably to our hearts.

A multitasker for heart health Research into the heart-protecting benefits of fish oil shows that it guards your ticker in a variety of ways. When we eat fish, omega-3s accumulate in cell membranes, where they help to:

- Normalize the heart's rate when outside influences try to make it skip a beat
- Slow the racing heartbeat that causes life-threatening ventricular fibrillation
- Prevent blood clots
- Slow the growth of plaque in arteries
- Lower triglyceride levels
- Strengthen blood vessels' walls

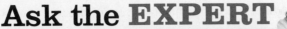

Ask the EXPERT

Samantha B. Cassetty, M.S., R.D.
Nutrition Director, GHRI

Q *How do I get omega-3s if I have a seafood allergy?*

Samantha says: There's some debate about whether fish oil supplements are OK for people with food allergies, but since no one knows for sure, I suggest you play it safe and steer clear of them. That leaves you with plant-based sources of omega-3s, like walnuts and canola oil. Although they don't have the same health benefits as fish fats, they do have anti-aging perks of their own. New research suggests that eating a Mediterranean-based diet that includes walnuts (very similar in spirit to the 7 Years Younger Meal Plan) is linked to a lower risk of heart attacks and strokes. Flaxseeds and chia seeds are other great sources of plant-based omega-3s. You can also pick up 500-mg supplements of algae-based DHA—one of the healthy fats found in fish. Since these are made from algae and not fish, they're considered safe for people with seafood allergies.

- Keep blood thin

The feel-full factor People who eat even the fattiest fish typically eat less red meat. Scientists theorize that this is the reason they generally have healthier hearts and slimmer bodies. But fatty fish, because of its oil, is generally higher in calories than leaner varieties, so how can it help keep you svelte? One study, involving 232 overweight volunteers on a reduced-calorie diet, set out to find the answer. The researchers discovered that when the dieters ate a meal that included a fatty fish, such as salmon, they felt fuller longer than those who ate a leaner fish, such as cod. It appears that high levels of omega-3s prompt the body to produce more leptin, the hormone that signals fullness. This, in turn, helps you eat less food throughout the day, the scientists hypothesize. Other studies suggest that omega-3 fatty acids may help block fat-cell formation.

A possible cancer fighter Does eating fish help reduce the risk of cancer, or is the rate of cancer low among fish eaters because they consume less red meat? It's a scientific conundrum, but there is evidence suggesting that eating a few servings of fish a week may offer protection against certain types of cancer, most notably colorectal cancer. In one study, European researchers spent five years following the dietary habits of patients admitted to the hospital for precancerous and cancerous polyps. They found that the risk increased with meat consumption and was "significantly reduced" with moderate fish intake, which was defined as one to two servings a week.

Protection from the sun Three British studies found that high levels of omega-3s in the diet helped protect people from sunburn. Studies in mice suggest how this can happen. When scientists exposed mice to ultraviolet radiation, they found that omega-3s significantly reduced inflammation and other immunological responses that break down collagen, which is vital to firm, youthful skin.

Mind sharpener Yes, it's true: Eating fish is good for the brain. A European study involving 2,031 elderly men and women found that those who regularly ate seafood performed better on cognitive tests than those who

Supplemental Protection

The *7 Years Younger Anti-Aging Breakthrough Diet* provides you with all the nutrients you need. Generally speaking, no nutritional supplements are necessary to safeguard your health, with two possible exceptions: fish oil and vitamin D. If you don't eat fish, health experts recommend taking 500 mg per day of supplemental fish oil (omega-3 fatty acids) containing both EPA and DHA. People with heart disease should aim for 800 to 1,000 mg per day. As for vitamin D, it's nearly impossible to get as much as you need from food. The official daily requirement for adults is 600 IU, but many health experts recommend 1,000 IU a day.

ate little or none.

What you'll eat You don't have to add a ton of seafood to your diet in order to enjoy the benefits of a fish-friendly diet. The 7 *Years Younger Anti-Aging Breakthrough Diet* offers just what the AHA recommends: fish at least twice a week.

Grains: Whole Ones Reign

Eating whole grains goes a long way toward keeping age-related disease at bay. Research conducted at the University of Scranton measured the polyphenol content of whole-grain flours and ready-to-eat whole-grain foods and snacks. Breakfast cereals (particularly whole-grain cold cereals) and popcorn topped the list, with an antioxidant content comparable to that of fruits and vegetables. Whole-grain flours such as those used to make whole wheat bread scored high, too. Overall, whole-grain foods had significantly more antioxidants than ones made from processed grains.

Feel-full foods Whole grains work doubly hard by keeping blood sugar levels steady and making you feel full longer. A research review of diet-friendly foods, including whole wheat versions of products like bread, pasta, and crackers as well as oats and brown rice, found that a menu loaded with whole grains helps people stay slim. One reason? Whole grains rank low on the glycemic index, a system that rates the effects of different carbohydrates on blood sugar levels, while refined grains rise to the top of the index. Researchers in Denmark followed 548 people who were on a low-fat maintenance program for eight weeks after they had lost an average of 24 pounds. Those who ate few refined grains and more lean meat, nuts, low-fat dairy, and whole grains—the foods found on the 7 *Years Younger Anti-Aging Breakthrough Diet*—didn't gain back any weight. However, those who ate high on the glycemic index—white bread and other refined carbohydrates—regained almost four pounds. When researchers from Tufts University analyzed the dietary habits of 434 men and women, they

Fill Up on Fiber

Fiber deserves special attention as an anti-aging superstar. It's found mainly in fruits, vegetables, whole grains, and beans–pillars of the *7 Years Younger Anti-Aging Breakthrough Diet*. Although the distinction isn't always apparent on a food label, there are two types of fiber: insoluble and soluble. Most fiber-rich foods contain both types–the insoluble kind helps improve your digestion, and the soluble kind gives fiber its disease-fighting clout. Fiber has these health pluses:

- **Shrinks belly fat** Soluble fiber, in particular, helps whittle your waist.

- **Controls cholesterol** Oats, beans, and other sources of soluble fiber help reduce LDL cholesterol, too much of which ratchets up your risk of heart attack.

- **Lowers heart disease risk** Fiber helps reduce blood pressure and disease-promoting inflammation.

- **Improves insulin sensitivity** The fiber in whole grains works even harder than the fiber in fruits and vegetables because it slows the absorption of sugar, making it easier for insulin to do its job.

- **Reduces cancer risk** When researchers looked at the fiber consumption of 35,972 women, they found that a diet rich in fiber from whole grains and fruit offered premenopausal women significant protection against breast cancer.

- **Aids in weight loss** One explanation: High-fiber foods take a long time to chew, giving your body time to send "I'm full" signals to the brain before you've overeaten. These foods also tend to take up space in your stomach, so you're likely to stay full for longer periods of time.

Just because a label boasts that a food has a high fiber content doesn't mean you'll reap all of these benefits. That's because many packaged foods are filled with supplemental fibers, including inulin, corn fiber, and polydextrose, which don't have all of the proven benefits of the fiber found naturally in foods. And these ingredients are more likely to cause gas and bloating.

Americans get only about 15 grams of fiber a day, not even close to the 25 grams recommended by the American Heart Association. But between whole grains, fruits and vegetables, beans, and nuts, you'll be exceeding that recommendation on the *7 Years Younger Anti-Aging Breakthrough Diet*.

Ask the EXPERT

Samantha B. Cassetty, M.S., R.D.
Nutrition Director, GHRI

Q *Does diet soda fit into the plan?*

Samantha says: Yes. Some research calls into question whether diet sodas help with weight loss, but that's partly because people who drink diet beverages may have an otherwise unhealthy diet (fast food, sweets, and salty snacks). On the 7 Years Younger Meal Plan, you'll be making healthy improvements to your diet, and ditching sugary sodas is one of those. Sugar is a skin ager, and regular soft drinks are loaded with it (and high in calories). That's why it's better to go with diet versions. If you prefer not to drink them, you can stick with water, seltzer, or unsweetened iced tea.

Q *I want to limit my sugar intake, but I love sweet things. Is it OK to use artificial sweeteners in my coffee and tea?*

Samantha says: I let the health authorities be my guide, and the FDA considers both artificial sweeteners and natural ones, like stevia, safe for most people (the exception: those with a rare metabolic disorder called phenylketonuria; they need to steer clear of aspartame). I'm also swayed by the National Cancer Institute's findings that there's no clear evidence that FDA-approved zero-calorie sweeteners are linked to cancer. Sugar, however, is linked to health problems, so I suggest cutting way back on it, including natural forms like maple syrup, honey, and agave. That includes sugar in your coffee and tea, so if you like your sips sweet, I'd suggest using a zero-calorie alternative. You'll notice that on the 7 Years Younger Meal Plan, we stick to small amounts of added sugar—no more than a teaspoon to sweeten yogurt, for instance—but we also include foods with noncaloric sweeteners. Since the plan is so flexible, the choice is yours.

found that those who ate about three servings of whole grains a day, mainly from cereal, had lower body mass indexes than those who ate less (25.4, versus 27.3). Even more important: They had 5% less belly fat.

Whole grains = healthier hearts Studies show a relationship between consumption of whole grains and a lower risk of cardiovascular disease. The ongoing Nurses' Health Study, for example, showed that after 10 years, nurses who ate whole grains, including dark bread, brown rice, popcorn, and whole-grain breakfast cereals, had a 30% lower risk of heart disease than those who ate refined-grain products such as white bread.

A study of 43,000 men showed results similar to those in the study of nurses. Those who ate the most whole grains were 30% less likely to develop heart disease.

Blood pressure reducers People with high blood pressure were able to bring it down by eating between 7.2 and 18.9 grams of wheat fiber a day, according to the findings from a number of studies conducted by researchers at Tulane University in New Orleans.

Cancer fighters Cancer risk drops as consumption of whole grains rises, according to a scientific review of 16 years' worth of studies involving

Dieter's Top Tip
The Beauty of the Benefits

Melissa Berman followed the 7 Years Younger Meal Plan precisely, and the payoff was amazing. After seven weeks, she dropped 19 pounds and 6½ inches from her 5'4" frame. She was rewarded in other ways, too. "I have more energy, I sleep better, my hair is full and looks shinier, and my skin looks healthier," says Melissa, who'd been wanting to lose her "baby fat" since she gave birth to her firstborn 11 years ago. "My pores are smaller, and my complexion is more even-toned."

She's convinced that it's all because she stuck closely to the daily meal and snack plan. "I wanted to get the maximum nutrition out of the diet, and it really paid off," she says.

20 kinds of cancer. This effect was most notable for colorectal cancer. Conversely, researchers also observed that diets containing refined grains led to increased cancer risk.

Skin savers Whole grains can brighten the complexion. "Refined grains can raise insulin levels, which in turn causes inflammation that damages the skin," says Adam Friedman, M.D., director of dermatologic research at Albert Einstein College of Medicine.

Whole grains are a good source of selenium, a mineral that helps protect skin against injury from ultraviolet rays. Beyond the beauty-related payoffs, a study conducted by Dutch and Australian researchers found that a high blood level of selenium was associated with around a 60% lowering of the incidence of non-melanoma skin cancer.

What you'll eat You'll meet your whole-grain quota by eating whole wheat breads, cereals, crackers, and pasta in lieu of white versions, but you'll also explore other whole grains including oats, brown rice, quinoa, and bulgur.

Legumes: Beans at Any Meal

Lowly legumes—beans, lentils, peas, and peanuts—are an inexpensive commodity, but they are priceless when it comes to your health. Beans are a rare source of vegetable protein. Substitute them for meat in meals, and you'll lower your intake of saturated fat, a notorious aging agent.

Belly-fat targeters Beans are nutritional fountains of youth. They are a great weight-loss food because they contain no saturated fat, making them an ideal substitute for red meat. However, their true contribution to weight loss comes from soluble fiber, which studies show can help reduce belly fat.

Cholesterol clobberers Studies have found that eating beans regularly can bring down total cholesterol and triglycerides. One study found that eating a half-cup of pinto beans a day can potentially slash "bad" LDL cholesterol by 8% or more in eight weeks. Every 1% drop in LDL can lower heart disease risk up to 3%; that makes a strong case for eating more beans.

A way to keep blood sugar steady Beans and lentils are among the high-fiber foods that get credit for keeping blood sugar stable. In one study, researchers compared two groups of people with type 2 diabetes after filling their diets with different amounts of fiber. One group ate the standard recommended diet of 25 grams of fiber per day, and the other group ate twice the fiber. The result: The higher-fiber group had better blood sugar levels and improved insulin sensitivity.

Cancer fighters Beans contain saponins, phytonutrients that inhibit cancer-cell production in lab tests. In one experiment at Michigan State University, a diet high in beans prevented the development of colon cancer in test animals injected with cancer-causing substances.

What you'll eat Kidney beans, Great Northern beans, chickpeas, and lentils—these are just some of the bean varieties you'll sample; whether they are already a staple of your diet or you're working them in for the first time, you're bound to discover new ways to enjoy legumes when you follow the 7 Years Younger Meal Plan.

STEER CLEAR: 7 YEARS YOUNGER ANTI-AGING BREAKTHROUGH DIET BUSTERS

Though there are many amazing foods in the culinary world that can aid you in reaching your health goals, there are three main things that can actually make you age faster: sugar, saturated fat, and alcohol. You should aim to keep these to a minimum, which we've done on the 7 Years Younger Anti-Aging Breakthrough Diet.

Sugar The average American woman consumes 18 teaspoons of added sugar (sugars and syrups that are added to foods during processing or preparation, including those added at the table) per day, and men consume an average of 26. That's a disaster if you're trying to lose weight. Sugar offers virtually nothing nutritional and wreaks havoc with your insulin levels, which in turn can send you false hunger signals. That's why it's enemy number one in the fight against diabetes. Also, when blood glucose goes up, this increases the creation of advanced glycation end products, which go by the appropriate acronym AGEs. AGEs take a toll on skin by interfering with the normal repair of collagen and of elastin, a protein that allows skin to get back its shape after stretching or contracting.

We eat about three and a half times as much sugar as we should, according to the American Heart Association, which recommends a limit of 6¼ teaspoons (about 100 calories' worth) per day to manage weight and reduce the risk of heart disease. (Sugars that are found naturally in foods, such as those in fruit, are OK.) Make a habit of reading labels: Even healthy products can be loaded with sugar, so be sure to steer away from foods that contain an added sugar as one of the first

5 Best and Worst Foods

When Harvard researchers analyzed dietary patterns and on-the-scale ups and downs of more than 120,000 men and women, they were able to single out specific foods contributing to the 3.4 pounds the average American gains over a four-year stretch. The "bad guys":

- Potato chips
- French fries
- Sugar-sweetened drinks
- Red and processed meats

The same report also included foods associated with weight loss. The "good guys":

- Fruits
- Nuts
- Vegetables
- Whole grains
- Yogurt

Sugar Shock: How Much Is Too Much?

It's all too easy to reach your daily limit of six teaspoons (about 25 grams) of added sugar—even when you skip dessert. That's why you need to read food labels. (Note: Labels show total sugars, which includes naturally occuring ones like lactose in dairy products.) Here, see how you can save 18¼ teaspoons of added sugar just by being smart about what you put in your cart.

Too Sweet   **Just Right**

	Product*	Tsp. Sugar	Cal.	Product*	Tsp. Sugar	Cal.
Breakfast	Cascadian Farm Dark Chocolate Almond Granola	3½	210	Fiber One Chocolate Flavored Cereal	1½	80
	Arnold 100% Whole Wheat Bread	1	220	Arnold Sandwich Thins	½	100
Lunch	Butterball Honey Roasted Turkey Breast	¾	60	Butterball Deli Inspirations Oven Roasted Turkey Breast	0	50
	B&G Sweet Pickles	1¾	35	B&G Kosher Baby Dill Gherkins	0	0
Snack	Snackwell's White Fudge Drizzled Caramel Popcorn	5	130	Angie's Boomchickapop Lightly Sweet Popcorn	1¼	120
	Sweet Baby Ray's Hickory & Brown Sugar Barbecue Sauce	4	70	McCormick Grill Mates Applewood Rub	¼	15
Dinner	B&M Vegetarian Baked Beans	3	160	Goya dark kidney beans	½	90
	Jiffy Corn Muffin (as prepared)	1¾	170	Bob's Red Mill Polenta Corn Grits	0	130
	Ken's Steak House French with Applewood Smoked Bacon Dressing	2¼	140	Ken's Steak House Russian Dressing	¾	140
Total	**Too Sweet**	**23**	**1,195**	**Just Right**	**4¾**	**725**

Sugar and calorie totals based on manufacturers' serving sizes.

three ingredients.

When reading labels, be aware that total sugar on the label does not refer only to added sugar. It also includes the natural sugars, such as those found in yogurt and juice. Sugars can be as well-disguised on labels as they are in foods. Any ingredient that contains the words "syrup" or "sweetener" or any word ending in "-ose" is a tip-off that the product contains sugar.

Saturated fat Beyond its nefarious reputation for clogging our arteries, the type of fat found in marbled meats and full-fat dairy products contributes to making you look older. "Eating a lot of saturated fat induces skin-aging inflammation," says Jane Grant-Kels, M.D., chair of dermatology at the University of Connecticut in Farmington. In addition, clogged arteries can negatively affect sexual health and cause memory problems.

Alcohol We're not saying you need to push away the wine list forever or resign yourself to water during happy hour. In fact, many studies suggest that light to moderate drinkers have a lower risk of cardiovascular disease and can have lower rates of certain cancers, heart disease, and even cog-

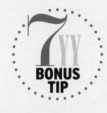

Oil Is Better Than Butter

Even if you don't save on calories, ditching butter for a drizzle of olive oil is a smart move. The fat facts: Scientists put 20 people with big bellies on a diet high in either saturated fat (the kind found in butter and other animal products) or monounsaturated fat (the kind found in olive, avocado, and nut oils). Saturated fats, the researchers learned, can cause disease-promoting inflammation. Monounsaturated ones, on the other hand, help fend off diabetes and heart disease and other ills associated with abdominal flab.

Ask the EXPERT

Samantha B. Cassetty, M.S., R.D.
Nutrition Director, GHRI

Q *I'm trying to eat gluten-free. How can I make this plan work?*

Samantha says: You're in luck! Many of the foods that are staples of the 7 Years Younger Meal Plan—things like fresh fruits and vegetables; lean meat, poultry, and fish; eggs; nuts; beans; and low-fat dairy products—are already gluten-free. When recipes call for pasta, substitute one made with whole-grain brown rice. Quinoa, another gluten-free grain, works well in dishes that call for couscous or bulgur (be wary of quinoa pastas, though, since they're made predominantly from corn). Fortunately, it's easy to find gluten-free versions of staples like bread and crackers at chain supermarkets. One caution about them: They often contain more calories and refined grains than traditional products, so read labels carefully and adjust your portions as needed.

Keep Yourself Hydrated

Staying hydrated is the key to having clear, radiant, and plump skin cells. If you're not drinking enough water, or if you're taking in too many dehydrating caffeinated beverages, your skin can look depleted and dull. Here's a quick fix: Swap your diet sodas and iced coffees for a cup of peppermint tea, hot or cold. Its anti-inflammatory properties can do wonders for the skin, and you should start seeing its skin-brightening effects in a week or less.

There is no specific rule for the amount of water you should drink every day, especially because you will also get water from the fruits and vegetables you eat. If you keep a beverage handy at most times, though, it's more likely that you'll stay completely hydrated and feeling good.

nitive decline. But excessive alcohol consumption can have a real effect on your weight management. Drinking on an empty stomach can lead you to eat more indulgently than you would otherwise, and alcohol itself adds calories to your day while doing nothing to appease your hunger. And the calorie count might surprise you: An ounce of 80-proof alcohol contains 90 calories. In terms of specific drinks, a five-ounce Bloody Mary could contain about 120 calories, depending on how it's made; a four-ounce Cosmopolitan could be around 200 calories, while eight ounces of a frosty piña colada could set you back a whopping 650 calories.

Beyond its possibly unexpected calories, alcohol can have other side effects. If you've ever experienced that dry-mouthed desperate-for-water awakening, you'll know that alcohol is dehydrating even if you haven't had enough to produce a hangover. Alcohol consumption can take a toll on your skin, making it dry, taut, and lined. Also, as the liver metabolizes alcohol, it creates free radicals, those other enemies of firm, youthful skin. Both women and men can enjoy a drink per day on the 7 *Years Younger Anti-Aging Breakthrough Diet* (once on maintenance, men can have two).

Activate Your Anti-Aging Diet Now!

1 **Fill your plate with a rainbow of colors** Age-reversing nutrients are found in foods that are red, orange, yellow, purple, blue, green... all hues. So eat up!

2 **Avoid youth-robbing foods** Sugar, alcohol, and refined-grain foods such as white bread, rice, and pasta offer no health benefits and promote the aging of skin. Avoid them, or at the very least keep them to a minimum in your diet.

3 **Pick your proteins well** You can make a cheat sheet of delicious lean proteins that will save you a ton of calories for next time you're at the grocery or out to dinner.

For more expert anti-aging advice, get our free special report 50 Ways to Stress Less & Live Longer at 7yearsyounger.com/stressless.

Chapter 2

Eat to Win-Win

Think of the *7 Years Younger Anti-Aging Breakthrough Diet* as a blueprint for a new you—a few sizes smaller and looking and feeling years younger, with firmer muscles and glowing skin. It's a delicious and nutritious plan that is low in calories without being skimpy on food. Hunger is not a problem on the *7 Years Younger Anti-Aging Breakthrough Diet*—and we have a group of dieters to prove it!

Every single one of our test panelists lost weight, most at a higher rate than the average half-pound to one pound per week generally lost on other calorie-counting programs. The meal plan not only helped keep their hunger at bay, but also actually boosted their energy.

Many people envision a healthy weight-loss diet as a time-consuming, restrictive way of eating that involves hard-to-find and, for some people, unappealing foods. Not *this* diet. The *7 Years Younger Anti-Aging Breakthrough Diet* is all about taste, with emphasis on ease and convenience.

There is no counting of calories or figuring out what you should eat, because we've done all the work for you. All you have to do is follow the plan meal by meal from day to day and you'll see the pounds and inches melt away. No, we are not kidding!

"At first I was skeptical that I could just eat these meals without having to count something, but it's so true how easy it is," says Melissa Berman, a stay-at-home mom who dropped 19 pounds in seven weeks, "without even feeling like I was trying."

"The diet is well balanced where you feel you are eating enough food and it gives you plenty of energy," says Robin Greenberg, a stay-at-home mom of three kids who lost 3½ pounds. "It is more of a lifestyle change than a diet." How's that for inspiration?

Next to taste, variety is the power behind the stick-to-itiveness of the *7 Years Younger Anti-Aging Breakthrough Diet*. You'll get to sample nearly 100 different foods, so monotony will never be an issue. There are plenty of food favorites, too—tacos, bagels, and even steak and fries—and an array of cuisines. Maybe you'll eat Mexican tonight and try Asian tomorrow. Is the family hankering for a trip to the pizza parlor? Well, you'll get to go and even enjoy the pizza, too. Fine dining on the agenda? We offer you plenty of tips so you can make the night deliciously extra special because you won't be "blowing" your diet or seeing the number on the scale creep back up the next day.

"The *7 Years Younger Anti-Aging Breakthrough Diet* is simply the easiest diet I've ever been on," says Michele Fredman, 61, a lawyer who lost 7½ pounds in seven weeks. Michele came to the *7 Years Younger Anti-Aging Breakthrough Diet* after having tried a variety of diets over the decades that she felt were too difficult or complicated to follow. "It doesn't even feel like a diet," she says of this one.

"This is the first diet I've ever been on that doesn't feel like a diet," agrees Carol Scudder-Danilowicz. "I was afraid I'd feel deprived, but instead I feel empowered and satisfied."

That's the whole idea. This is not a weight-loss diet that you go on and off of. Rather, it is a new way of eating, one designed to put you on a healthy track forever. It means losing weight gradually—and, most important, permanently. It's all about embarking on a new healthy lifestyle, one built around the foods that will continually nurture you from the inside out, the foods that will make you grow younger as you get thinner. On the 7 Years Younger Meal Plan, you'll be eating age-defying foods at every meal. It's how you'll recapture the youthful glow you thought vanished along with your waistline. Not only will you look great because you're eating well, but you'll look younger, because your new style of eating includes foods that have anti-aging and skin-enhancing properties—a rainbow of colorful vegetables, fruits, legumes, and whole grains you'll be reaching for every day.

Planning your daily meals and snacks around these foods means you'll be eating items that are naturally low in calories and high in nutrients. You won't get between-meals hunger because you'll be eating the right amount of fat, protein, and fiber at each meal to make you feel fuller longer. You won't have to think about how to fit the right amount of skin-protecting and age-reversing foods into your day or worry about counting calories at each meal, because we've done it all for you and packaged it into a 7 Years Younger Meal Plan—the backbone of the diet.

Best of all, the *7 Years Younger Anti-Aging Breakthrough Diet* is designed to include everyone's favorite foods and to fit into any lifestyle, whether you have to please finicky kids, you're cooking for one or two (you and the "thin one"), or you're on the road and forced to eat out five days a week. Everyone will reap the healthful benefits, even those for whom weight loss isn't a priority. If you have kids, think of this diet as an investment in their futures. Studies show that when kids learn healthy eating habits at a young age, those habits are established for a lifetime.

Daniel Chin
"I had faith
in the
information"

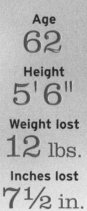

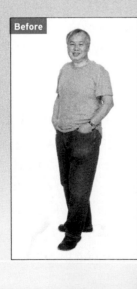

Before

Age
62

Height
5'6"

Weight lost
12 lbs.

Inches lost
7½ in.

STRUGGLES IN PAST DIETING HISTORY "Prior diets had less variety and quality of meal offerings and were too rigid."

WHY 7YY "I had faith in the fact that the information and meals were developed and tested by the Good Housekeeping Research Institute."

SUCCESS SECRET "I learned two really important tricks: portion control and switching from white rice to brown rice and from regular pasta to whole wheat. You just don't realize how many calories you eat day after day when you don't pay attention to it. My wife and I were totally out of touch with portion control." (See Gean Chin on page 80.)

PROUDEST OF "[The fact that] a large part of my success was achieved by keeping portions under control and not eating until completely full."

FAVORITE 7YY RECIPE "Ziti with Peas, Grape Tomatoes & Ricotta [page 246] and Spice-Rubbed Pork Tenderloin [page 261]. "

BEST ADVICE FOR OTHER DIETERS "The 7 *Years Younger Anti-Aging Breakthrough Diet* really works, and your results will be a function of how disciplined you can be about staying on the plan. Even though I strayed from the plan at times during the seven weeks, I still was able to achieve a decent weight loss that I'm proud of."

Now that you know about all these great possibilities, let's find out the healthy and delicious ways you're going to enjoy them, just as our panelists did. The *7 Years Younger Anti-Aging Breakthrough Diet* thwarts hunger by zeroing in on nutrient-dense calories strategically proportioned into this daily formula:

- 25% protein
- 50% carbohydrates
- 25% fat, with only 7% coming from saturated fat

"Nutrient-dense" means you get filling foods so you won't end up famished, and the variety of foods offered on this diet means you won't get bored, which will also diminish cravings. It means you'll be eating real meals—full and satisfying ones—not the mini meals suggested by so many other diets. Mini meals don't work in the long haul because they put you out of sync with how the rest of the world lives and eats.

The 3-4-5 Solution

The slenderizing, skin-nourishing anti-aging nutrients in the *7 Years Younger Anti-Aging Breakthrough Diet* are packed into an exclusive easy-to-follow 3-4-5 Plan—300 calories for breakfast, 400 calories at lunch, and a 500-calorie dinner. This keeps your calorie intake high enough that you won't feel hungry, but low enough to facilitate weight loss. You don't have to remember the formula or worry about hitting the right numbers, because the meal plans that we've created do those things for you. The 3-4-5 Plan aligns with how people typically eat their way through the day, ending with the largest meal. In addition, after the Jumpstart week that kicks off and turbocharges the plan, there are 250 calories' worth of snacks for women and between 350 and 500 calories' worth of snacks for men. (Pound for pound, men need more calories than women because they typically have more lean tissue, or muscle, which burns calories more efficiently.) It all adds up to a daily total of:

- 1,450 calories for women;
- 1,575 calories for slightly to moderately active men (which includes most men);
- 1,700 calories for highly active men, meaning those who have labor-intensive jobs or who work out a good hour a day about five times a week.

There's room for two snacks a day, one in mid-afternoon and the other in the evening. Snacking is important because it staves off hunger when you go long hours between meals. Generally speaking, you shouldn't go more than three hours without food from the time you get up in the morning until your last meal of the day. This means most people don't need a mid-morning snack, but they do need one in the afternoon. There's also room for a second snack after dinner.

The 3-4-5 Plan can be personalized to accommodate an on-the-go lifestyle. There are options for dining out or popping a meal in the microwave. And check out the easy recipes on pages 281–291 based on a supermarket rotisserie chicken, whole wheat pasta, or canned tuna or beans.

One thing to remember, though: The 3-4-5 Plan is designed to deliver satisfaction at every meal of every day, so no borrowing calories from one meal to save up so you can eat more at another. Cutting back on calories at a meal will make you more likely to be starving by the time the next one rolls around. That weakens your willpower and puts you at risk of going off the plan. Give yourself a fair shot and try to stick closely to the recommendations (see "Ask the Expert," page 69, for more on this topic).

Seven Weeks of Delicious Menus

The 7 *Years Younger Anti-Aging Breakthrough Diet*'s exclusive 7 Years Younger Meal Plan is the model for the way you'll want to eat for the rest of your life—a diet based on the foods that will keep your weight in check, keep your skin firm and glowing, and help fight age-related diseases. Eat from it each day at each meal, and you will learn how to judge what a serving should be whether you're eating at home, taking the family to a fast-food chain, or joining friends for happy hour. "This diet's given me more energy," says Lynn Bunis, a 54-year-old school administrator who wanted to find a diet that worked after realizing she was buying clothes to hide rather than accentuate her figure. After losing

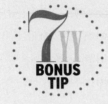

Nuts: The Super Snack

Nuts and seeds generally are not considered a "diet food" because they are high in calories, but they play an important role in both helping you lose weight and keeping your skin vibrant. It doesn't take a lot—less than a handful a day—to reap the benefits, so don't pass up nuts as a nutritious snack because of their calories. Nut eaters weigh, on average, 4 pounds less than people who munch on other types of snacks, according to one study. The reason? People find nuts filling, which can stop them from going to other snacks that aren't as filling. Best of all, up to 20% of the calories in nuts don't get absorbed.

Research shows that people who eat nuts at least five times a week live longer than people who eat them infrequently. A major study on the Mediterranean diet involving more than 7,000 people found that people who ate on average an ounce of nuts a day had a "significant" 30% reduction in their risk of stroke.

If you are wondering how many nuts you can eat in one protein-packed 125-calorie snack, here's the scoop:

- 9 walnut halves
- 17 almonds
- 30 pistachios
- 13 cashews
- 23 peanuts

14 pounds and 7½ inches in seven weeks, she said, "I am sleeping better and have more energy. I feel a bounce in my step when I walk to work that I haven't felt in a long time."

Week 1 is intended to give you a good jumpstart, so we've left snacks out of the first seven days, the time when motivation is at its highest. Our panelists reported having no trouble skipping snacks the first week. In fact, many of them were so delighted with their first week's weight loss and their lack of hunger or cravings, they asked if they could continue eliminating snacks. A second week without snacks may be OK for the truly motivated, but ideally you should eat the snacks recommended in the plan. Why? Because they are part of the master plan to deliver maximum anti-aging nutrition. They also go a long way toward filling you up and staving off between-meals hunger.

The meals and the snacks built into each day and each week were carefully designed and calibrated for calories and key nutrients by the Good Housekeeping Research Institute's nutrition director, Samantha Cassetty, M.S., R.D., to maximize the 7 *Years Younger Anti-Aging Breakthrough Diet's* unique pound-dropping, anti-aging formula. By following the 7 Years Younger Meal Plan, you are guaranteed to get:

Dieter's Top Tip

Protein Has Power

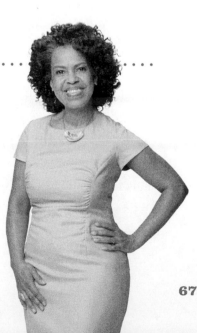

As a proponent of holistic health, book editor Malaika Adero, 56, knows a lot about healthy eating, but what she didn't know about was the power of eating protein at every meal. "Eating a little protein in a meal does help stop hunger pangs. It really works!" says Malaika, who lost 8 pounds in seven weeks.

Five to seven ounces of animal protein plus the equivalent from other protein sources, such as beans, seeds, nuts, eggs, and soy, every day You'll get to savor some at every meal, from Smoked-Salmon Scrambled Eggs (page 227) and Ham & Veggie Hash (page 225) at breakfast to Chicken Caesar Pitas (page 234) and Spicy Black Bean Soup (page 239) at lunch to Beef Ragu (page 262) and Orange Pork & Asparagus Stir-Fry (page 259) at dinner. **The equivalent of two to three servings of dairy per day** A serving is a cup of low-fat or fat-free milk or yogurt or an ounce of cheese, though you may not get a full serving at every meal. Fitting dairy into your day can be much more interesting than just pouring skim milk over your cereal. You can start out the day with milk blended in our satisfying Banana–Peanut Butter Smoothie (page 223), or with the luscious part-skim ricotta in the Sweet Stuffed Waffle (page 222)—one of our panelists' favorite recipes based on how tasty it was. You could enjoy the Grilled Mozzarella & Tomato Soup (page 229) or end the day with the cheesy Big Fusilli Bowl (page 242) at dinner. Cheese is a popular food that tends to be high in calories, and our recipes demonstrate how a little can go a very satisfyingly long way.

Two to five servings of fruit per day A serving is considered a medium piece of whole fruit or about a cup of sliced or diced fruit, and you'll find

Fruit Swaps

You can swap any of the fruits in our meal plan for other choices. Here's a calorie guide to easy-to-fit-in-and-swap-out snacks:

50 calories
- 1 cup blueberries
- 1 cup cantaloupe chunks
- ½ grapefruit
- 1 cup honeydew melon chunks
- 1 kiwifruit
- 1 small orange
- 1 cup raspberries
- 15 strawberries

100 calories
- 1 medium apple
- 1 medium banana
- 1 cup cherries
- 1 cup grapes
- 1 small pear

Ask the EXPERT

Samantha B. Cassetty, M.S., R.D.
Nutrition Director, GHRI

Q *Let's say I want to have a beer and a few nachos after work...does that replace dinner?*

Samantha says: Bar food isn't on the plan, so I can't give this one my blessing. A plate of nachos starts in the neighborhood of 1,500 calories and climbs from there. See if you can get by with a beer (about 100 calories for a bottle of a light variety) and one bite, and count it as a snack. Afterward, have a more sensible, balanced meal at home. If it's too tough to say, "No, thanks," count it as a dinner and then make a mental U-turn right back to the 7 Years Younger Meal Plan.

Q *I'm worried about overloading my system with all that fiber. Any tips on how to handle that?*

Samantha says: As healthy as they are, high-fiber foods like fruits, vegetables, whole grains, and beans are some of the worst triggers of, ahem, gas. Bloating and discomfort will ease up once your body gets used to eating these foods regularly, so the key is to introduce them gradually to let your system get accustomed to them. Since the 7 Years Younger Meal Plan is mapped out to provide lots of fiber, you can start by swapping a lower-fiber veggie, like zucchini, for a higher-fiber one, like broccoli. That will allow you to adapt to the numerous whole grains and beans on the plan. You can also try Beano; it's a natural enzyme available in a tablet (to chew or swallow) that, when taken with a meal, can help prevent gas. (Despite its name, Beano can be used not just with beans, but with any gas-producing food.)

It's a good idea to eliminate other causes of gas, too, such as chewing gum, smoking cigarettes, and eating foods made with sugar alcohols like sorbitol and maltitol (neither sugar nor alcohol, these reduced-calorie sweeteners get only partially absorbed; they're found in many sugar-free products). Also drink plenty of water and keep up your workouts—both can help ease any discomfort.

servings built in throughout the day—often in surprisingly decadent desserts. For example, Peach Melba Yogurt (page 222) is a fruity way to start the day, and cherries with a creamy wedge of goat cheese or Brie (Cherries & Cheese, page 278) make for a delicious snack. You can enjoy half a pear sprinkled with cinnamon and topped with crushed walnuts for a dessert with the Mediterranean Vegetarian Wrap (page 230) or an apple with the Protein Plate (page 231) for lunch. For dinner, you'll find fruit in meals such as the Pomegranate-Glazed Salmon (page 271) and Basil-Orange Chicken with Couscous (page 247).

Don't, however, discount an apple, an orange, a pear, or a piece of cantaloupe as a good idea for a snack or dessert. Eating plain fruit is an important way to get to five servings a day and a nutritious way to satisfy a sweet tooth.

Three to six servings of skin-enhancing, anti-aging, antioxidant-rich vegetables each day A serving is considered one-half cup, so you'll find antioxidant-rich greens and other colorful vegetables at almost every meal. Luckily, the 7 *Years Younger Anti-Aging Breakthrough Diet* makes it easy to sneak a serving or two into every entrée. Greens transform the common grilled cheese in our Open-Face Jarlsberg Sandwiches with Greens (page 237) and elevate the omelet to dinner status in our Garden-Vegetable Omelet (page 243). Watercress serves as a nutritious bed for Lemon-Mint Chicken Cutlets (page 255). Seared Salmon with Sweet Potatoes (page 274), a nutritional powerhouse on its own, gets an extra antioxidant kick when served on a bed of spinach. And there's even room for tomatoes and arugula in the Steak Sandwich with Grilled Onions (page 264).

Three to five servings of whole grains per day The 7 *Years Younger Anti-Aging Breakthrough Diet* makes delving into the wide world of grains more interesting than just eating a piece of whole-grain toast at breakfast or wrapping a whole-grain tortilla around your lunch fixings. Rice, couscous, pasta, waffles, noodles, and more are all part of the variety.

For example, you get your choice of using buckwheat soba noodles or whole wheat linguine in the Soba Noodle Bowl with Shrimp & Snow Peas (page 276). The crunch in the Crispy Fish Sandwiches (page 267) comes from real bread crumbs—and you even get a bun (whole wheat, naturally). You'll help meet your daily whole-grain requirement by adding whole wheat bread crumbs to Healthy-Makeover Meatloaf (page 254) and Chicken Parm Stacks (page 250). Yes, every little bit counts, because it all adds up throughout the day.

Learning all about the wide array of whole grains readily available in the marketplace was a delicious journey for many of our panelists—especially Gean and Daniel Chin, who went on the 7 *Years Younger Anti-Aging Breakthrough Diet* as a team. "We used to eat white rice almost every day...it's part of our culture," says Daniel. "We gradually migrated to whole grains, and now we've eliminated all the white carbs from our diet. Things like whole wheat, quinoa, and bulgur are now staples in our kitchen."

Fish twice a week The omega-3 fatty acids that are so important to heart health and dewy skin come primarily from fish, and you can get their

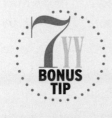

Popcorn: A Go-To Snack

Yes, it counts as a whole grain, but it only works as a smart weight-loss food if you're careful about how it's popped. Even a small bag of movie-theater popcorn can cost you 19 grams of saturated fat and 400 calories—and that's before you ask for melted-butter topping. Instead, keep a stash of microwavable kernels nearby to enjoy when you're looking for an afternoon treat—a bag of 94% fat-free microwave popcorn comes in at only 110 calories for four cups.

protective effects by eating fish twice a week. How do Scallop & Cherry Tomato Skewers (page 273), Shrimp & Fresh Corn Grits (page 275), and Tuna & Cannellini Bean Salad (page 241) sound? Our testers loved them all. Another fave: Shrimp Caesar Salad (page 232). You'll also find a number of different ways to enjoy salmon, including as a burger; as one of the richest sources of omega-3s that swim in the ocean, it's a great thing to include in your regular diet!

Avoid the coffee trap When it's served black, coffee is a zero-calorie beverage, but today's coffee industry has created a food group of its own, and many of the offerings are loaded with calories. A dizzying array of lattes and other coffee-related wake-up calls can be found just about everywhere—small or large, hot or cold, with mocha and with cream. It is possible to swallow your allotment of calories for a whole breakfast and possibly lunch before you even get to work. For example, the Venti Vanilla Frappuccino Blended Coffee with Whipped Cream at Starbucks is over 500 calories, and a large frozen Coffee Coolatta with Cream from Dunkin' Donuts is 860 calories.

If stopping for coffee is an important ritual for you, make it a point to know the calories in the cup before you take your first sip. And it's always best to check the nutritional analysis of your favorite brews. A cup of freshly brewed coffee at Starbucks, for example, has only 5 calories, but the innocuous-sounding iced coffee has 90 calories unless you ask the barista to hold the sweetener.

Built-In Flexibility

You'll lose weight the fastest, reap the most anti-aging benefits, and get the greatest grasp on how to make healthy eating and cooking a lifelong habit by following the 7 Years Younger Meal Plan exactly as it's designed. Follow it to a T, and you'll notice a surge in energy, your hair will be shinier, and your skin will be smoother. Maximum weight loss is virtually guaranteed.

However, the plan is not intended to be absolutely rigid. Flexibility is the beauty of the *7 Years Younger Anti-Aging Breakthrough Diet.*

We know what the real world is like because we listen to our readers—and we live in it ourselves. The simplicity of the 3-4-5 Plan means that

The Lowdown on Liquids

The best beverage for your calorie budget is water. Liquid calories simply aren't worth your while, because they do nothing to fill you up—the ultimate example of "empty calories"!

For example, an eight-ounce glass of apple juice is 114 calories, and it takes at least four apples, at 95 calories each, to extract that much liquid. **If you like the taste of apples, you're much better off eating the fruit.**

Can't imagine breakfast without orange juice? Just four ounces is 60 calories, about the same as eating an orange. But unless it's fresh-squeezed, the juice also could contain additives and preservatives, and four ounces won't be enough to last you through your whole meal! The orange, though, will last longer and offer more taste satisfaction.

The one exception to the juice rule is **vegetable juice: It may actually help you lose weight,** according to a study at Baylor College of Medicine. When researchers put 81 overweight people on a diet rich in fruits, vegetables, whole grains, and lean meats—the same foods found in the *7 Years Younger Anti-Aging Breakthrough Diet*—they found that those who drank an eight-ounce glass of low-sodium vegetable juice every day for three months lost on average three more pounds than those following the same diet without the juice. They theorized that the juice filled people up so they ate less overall. This kind of juice is so low in calories that it can fit quite easily into the 3-4-5 Plan without tipping the calorie scale. Eight ounces of low-sodium vegetable juice contain only 51 calories; the same amount of low-sodium tomato juice is 41 calories. Either one also counts for two servings of vegetables. Try sipping a glass while you are preparing dinner to help prevent pre-meal noshing and to boost your vegetable intake for the day.

meal options within a category are interchangeable. If, for example, you just aren't in the mood to make the Spice-Rubbed Pork Tenderloin (page 261) for dinner on Day 1 of Week 5, then swap it out for another dinner from our selection of recipes. There are 64 dinners to choose from, and they are all about 500 calories, so it's easy to substitute one for another. The same goes for the breakfasts and lunches. If Day 2's Sweet Stuffed Waffle (page 222) isn't your thing, then just swap it out for another breakfast. It's that easy!

In all, the 7 *Years Younger Anti-Aging Breakthrough Diet* offers 49 different daily nutrient-packed menus to choose from. If you're like our test panelists, you'll earmark your favorites as you work your way through the daily options so you can come back to them again and again. The emphasis on simplicity also means that all the meals and recipes featured in the 7 Years Younger Meal Plan are easy to prepare. You won't have to spend hours slicing and dicing; there are no 13-ingredient sauces to go with a 10-ingredient pasta, and there's no need to go from market to market in search of exotic foods. The recipes take about 30 minutes or less of hands-on time, and most of our breakfasts and lunches can be made in minutes.

"The menu plan is so much fun," says Leigh Gillam, 56, office manager for a home-care agency. "It doesn't get any easier than 300 calories at breakfast, 400 calories at lunch, and 500 calories at dinner. I've found that eating this way, I am not hungry like I used to be, especially after exercising." Leigh whittled off 12 pounds on the diet.

Fitting Convenience Into Your Diet

Part of our mission in creating this diet was to give you healthy choices everywhere you find yourself, including the fast-food line and the frozen-food aisle. While many experts these days frown on commercial products, fast food, and other convenience items, seeing them as being linked to obesity, there are good choices that can make your life easier.

On-the-Go Snacks
for Your Sweet Tooth

Have a hankering for a sweet treat other than the ones recommended on the plan? We scoured the market (both on foot and online) and narrowed our picks to goodies that have 125 calories or less—the same as our 7 Years Younger Meal Plan snacks—and no more than 7 grams of sugar. Then we let dozens of volunteers taste and weigh in with their thoughts. These dessert-worthy options were tops in our tests.

Kind Mini Fruit & Nut Delight
120 calories, 5 g sugar, 3 g protein, 2 g fiber
With "just the right amount of sweetness," this bar won praise for its "crunchy" texture and "whole nuts." (Only available online.)

Kellogg's FiberPlus Antioxidants Chocolate Chip
120 calories, 7 g sugar, 2 g protein, 9 g fiber
 "Lots of chocolate" sums up the praise for this "indulgent" treat that only "tastes unhealthy."

South Beach Diet Snack Bar in Fudgy Chocolate Mint
100 calories, 5 g sugar, 6 g protein, 6 g fiber
Tasters agreed that this snack reminded them of a Thin Mint Girl Scout cookie.

Special K Cereal Bar in Chocolatey Pretzel
90 calories, 6 g sugar, 1 g protein, 3 g fiber
The "salty-sweet combo" was deemed "soooo good."

Fiber One 90 Calorie Chocolate Peanut Butter Brownie
90 calories, 7 g sugar, 1 g protein, 5 g fiber
The "chewy," "cakelike" bar won many people over.

Kashi Dark Chocolate Coconut Layered Granola Bar
120 calories, 7 g sugar, 4 g protein, 4 g fiber
The "full-bodied chocolate taste" was a hit, as was the "real coconut."

7YY-Friendly Options From the Freezer Section

Frozen entrées serve as a form of enforced portion control: One box is usually one serving. "You don't have to measure, count, or weigh food to calculate the calories," says Dr. Bartfield of Loyola University Health Systems in Proviso, IL.

And the taste? With hundreds of products to choose from, we thought it was a good idea to help you out by sampling some of what's out there. Over the course of three weeks, testers in the the Good Housekeeping Research Institute rated nearly 400 boxes and steamer bags to come up with the tastiest options. Just keep in mind that none of these entrées have enough calories to fulfill the lunch or dinner calorie requirements, so you can round out these meals with healthy sides such as a serving of fruit or vegetables.

1. **Amy's Light & Lean Soft Taco Fiesta** *(220 calories)* This was rated number one because of its just-right spices. "Tastes like real Mexican takeout" was the overwhelming consensus.

2. **Amy's Light & Lean Spinach Lasagna** *(250 calories)* This came in second for its good taste and texture. Our tasters also appreciated its "nice portion size." Some people wished for a little more cheese.

3. **Amy's Light & Lean Pasta & Veggies** *(210 calories)* Though some complained about "too-soft noodles," the "crispy veggies" and "restaurant quality" earned high praise.

4. **Lean Cuisine Market Collection Chicken Poblano** *(300 calories)* Our tasters loved the chili-Cheddar sauce, though some wished there were more chicken.

5. **Healthy Choice 100% Natural Tortellini Primavera Parmesan** *(230 calories)* The "fresh" veggies won kudos from our tasters, as did the sauce. A few felt the portion size was a little small.

6 **Amy's Light & Lean Sweet & Sour Asian Noodle Bowl**
(250 calories) The ginger-and-garlic flavor got raves. Our tasters were pleased with how well the vegetables held up to microwaving.

7 **Healthy Choice 100% Natural Teriyaki Stir-Fry** *(250 calories)*
Tasters enjoyed the extras: "Pineapple and mushrooms were great additions." Some thought the sauce was a little sweet.

8 **Amy's Light & Lean Cheese Penne Marinara** *(270 calories)*
"Full of flavor" was the consensus, though some found the serving size a little small.

9 **Helen's Kitchen Veggie Fajita Bowl** *(250 calories)* The hearty portion and vegetable variety won praise, though some felt it "could use more seasoning."

10 **Amy's Light & Lean Spaghetti Italiano** *(240 calories)* The lentil-quinoa-tofu meatballs were a nice surprise for some non-vegetarians. Others found them "grainy."

11 **Amy's Light & Lean Bean & Cheese Burrito** *(280 calories)*
Bean lovers appreciated the abundance, though cheese fans were a bit disappointed. Some felt it was more of a snack than an entrée.

12 **Helen's Kitchen Fiesta Black Bean Bowl** *(290 calories)* The reviews on this ranged from "tastes as good as some real meals I've had" to "bland."

13 **Organic Bistro Sesame Ginger Wild Salmon Bowl**
(300 calories) Though tasters wished there were more sauce, this still got points for its "delicious" veggies and quinoa.

Ask the **EXPERT**

Samantha B. Cassetty, M.S., R.D.
Nutrition Director, GHRI

Q *Does the hour when I eat dinner matter? Is it true that the earlier you eat, the more you lose?*

Samantha says: Most dieters believe meal timing does count, but scientific evidence doesn't provide a clear yes or no. One recent study hinted that a group of Spanish people who ate a big midday meal lost more weight than those whose largest meal was a few hours later in the afternoon, but the results don't translate well in the United States, where we're used to eating our biggest meal in the evening. One thing is clear, though: People who eat more at night tend to snack their way through prime-time television, and they also tend to be breakfast skippers–two patterns that can make it hard to lose weight. Dinners on the 7 Years Younger Meal Plan are slightly bigger than lunches, a style of eating that matches how most of us dine. And although there's an evening snack, the calorie control and focus on the quality of the food you're eating will tip the scales in your favor–whether you're eating at 5 P.M. or 8 P.M.

Q *I'm not a fan of whole wheat bread or whole wheat pasta. What should I do?*

Samantha says: You're not alone. For many people, whole wheat products are an acquired taste. To make the switch, try some of the "soft" whole wheat varieties; their texture more closely matches the chewiness of white bread. And you may want to put Bella Terra Whole Wheat Penne on your shopping list: It rated tops in a GHRI taste test of whole wheat pastas for having a mild flavor that was "most similar to white pasta." If these options don't convert you, you can try a whole-grain blend–a product that contains a mixture of whole grains and refined ones. But since whole grains have fiber and other anti-aging nutrients, your goal should still be 100% whole grains.

The Good Housekeeping Research Institute has tasted and tested hundreds of convenience foods that stay true to our get-thinner, look-younger goal. Our menus and recipes take full advantage of these—a real time saver. But for when cooking isn't an option, we've also come up with the best frozen meals for the plan (see "7YY-Friendly Options From the Freezer Section," pages 76–77.) "The taste, nutrition, overall quality, and variety of frozen food have improved tremendously," says Jessica Bartfield, M.D., a nutrition and weight-management specialist at Loyola University Health Systems in Proviso, IL. According to several major studies, people who incorporated calorie-controlled convenience meals into their reducing strategy lost a "significant" percentage of their body weight. "I often recommend to my patients looking to lose weight that they fulfill at least one of the three basic meals with a frozen entrée as a proven dieting strategy," says Dr. Bartfield.

Moving Into Maintenance Mode

Remember how we said this is not the kind of diet you go on, then go off of? The 7 *Years Younger Anti-Aging Breakthrough Diet* is designed as an approach to eating that you will adopt for yourself and your family to serve you for a lifetime. Don't think of these nutrition recommendations as temporary; think of them as your new template for meal planning that will ensure that your body is getting everything it needs to remain healthy for the long term.

The 7 Years Younger Meal Plan is calibrated so that you'll get the right nutrition and number of calories every day. Once you're in maintenance mode, you can still calculate your ideal caloric intake in order to stay at your ideal weight. How do you know what your calorie limit should be? One option is to do the math. It takes about 15 calories a day to support one pound. If your ideal weight is, say, 140 pounds, you should be eating about 2,100 calories a day to sustain it. (The math: 140 x 15 = 2,100).

Gean Chin
"Be mindful
of what
you're
eating"

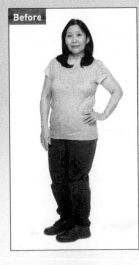

Before

Age
61

Height
5' 1¾"

Weight lost
6½ lbs.

Inches lost
6 in.

STRUGGLES IN PAST DIETING HISTORY "Not having a support group. Interacting with other dieters on Facebook helped keep me on track and was an encouragement for me to continue."

WHY 7YY "I wanted to lose weight and inches on a program that was healthy and would lead to making a lifelong change in the types of foods and the portion sizes I eat. My husband and I went on the program together so we could feel and look younger together and be supportive of each other." (See Daniel Chin on page 62.)

SUCCESS SECRET "Recording what I eat and keeping track of my calorie intake in a diet journal. Diet-wise, I made the switch to whole grains and now stay away from white carbs and fruit juices."

The Chins enjoy dining out, something they did not want to give up. They've just learned to do it differently. "When we eat in Chinatown, I push away the rice," says Gean. "If the food is fried, I take off the breading and just eat what's inside. When we go to a steak house, I cut the meat in half and have the other half packed up to take home. We say, 'No, thank you' to the bread the server brings."

PROUDEST OF "Getting into the habit of eating a healthy breakfast every day."

FAVORITE 7YY RECIPE "Easy Oatmeal [page 221] for breakfast, Veggie Burger [page 232] for lunch, and Seared Salmon with Sweet Potatoes [page 274] for dinner."

BEST ADVICE FOR OTHER DIETERS "Be mindful of what you're eating—chew your food more, and eat slowly. And keep walking!"

Want to be a panelist for a future 7 Years Younger plan? Sign up at 7yearsyounger.com/panelist to be considered.

Of course, this is only an approximation. There are a lot of variables—in particular, your activity level—that affect how many calories you burn in a day. If you're mostly sedentary, you might gain weight at 2,100 calories a day. If you walk or jog five miles a day, you may need more food. In the real world, the number of calories you need to sustain your ideal weight can vary even from day to day. The best solution: Make friends with your scale, and if you don't own a scale, get one. Weigh yourself daily, or at least two or three times a week. A fluctuation of three pounds from one day to the next is normal. However, if you see the scale hit five pounds above where you want to be, take it as a sign that you should look more closely at your eating over the last few weeks. It means that not only are you carrying around extra water weight, but you've likely also added some fat. So hop back on the Jumpstart Week 1 of the 7 Years Younger Meal Plan. A week, or possibly even two, on the plan should get you back where you want to be. And keep your food diary handy, too; going over the food journal you kept while losing weight should offer clues.

Changing your mindset about food in this way will help you stay focused on the priorities that will keep you looking and feeling great long past the first seven weeks. It will also give you the knowledge and confidence you need to navigate real-world situations that can feel like diet derailers. So if your spouse or friends are begging for a dine-out night, go

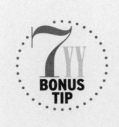

At the end of the seven weeks, you can loosen up on portion sizes a little or have an extra snack if you find yourself wanting one. See if your weight stays steady, you continue to lose, or you actually begin to regain weight. This, combined with looking at the trends on your scale, will help you figure out what and how you need to be eating in order to stay in maintenance mode.

for it! Remember, you're aiming to make healthy eating a lifestyle, and that means making sure to have fun! We give you details in Chapter 7 about how to avoid dining-out traps so that you can have a stress-free dining experience at various kinds of restaurants—yes, even fast-food places. Delicious, nutritious, and easy was our goal, and you'll find we live up to it all the way.

As you move on, you may not continue to eat the same meals and snacks you did when you were on the plan. But whatever you do, base your recipes on and choose your snacks and restaurant selections using the same foundation of lean, nutrient-rich anti-aging foods found in the 7 *Years Younger Anti-Aging Breakthrough Diet*. Keep an eye on the size of your plate for moderation and monitor the feeling of your stomach for satiety.

When you are deciding whether to indulge, ask yourself if the food is something you really want or if it's something you're choosing simply because it's available. Then ask yourself if you're really hungry or if you're just eating because the food is there or you want to be polite. As you'll learn as you read on, there is nothing rude about turning down food. Remember, it's not the last piece of cake or ice cream cone you'll ever be offered. Smile and just say, "No, thanks." You'll be glad you did when you step on the scale the next morning.

Smart Swaps

Just how badly do you want those pancakes or that piece of cheesecake? It pays—sometimes big-time—to know the calories in your favorite foods. Swapping a high-calorie item for something similar in taste can often appease your craving for the food. Our nutritionists swapped these 16 randomly selected items for something similar and came up with a total savings of 4,492 calories.

Swap this...	for this...	and save...
I order IHOP Cinn-A-Stack French Toast (1,120 cals)	2 Pillsbury Cinnamon Rolls with Icing (280 cals)	840 calories
1 slice Olive Garden White Chocolate Raspberry Cheesecake (890 cals)	1 Olive Garden Strawberry Mousse Dolcini dessert (210 cals)	680 calories
7 Buffalo wings with celery and blue cheese dressing (860 cals)	7½ oz. homemade chicken tenders (285 cals)	575 calories
Fast-food deluxe hamburger (710 cals)	Veggie burger (250 cals)	460 calories
1 bottle (about two servings) Naked Protein Zone Double Berry smoothie (440 cals)	1 bottle Dannon DanActive Blueberry Dairy Drink (70 cals)	370 calories
2 cups takeout Chinese fried rice (605 cals)	2 cups rice with steamed vegetables (300 cals)	305 calories
5 oz. fast-food french fries (450 cals)	5 oz. oven-baked fries (145 cals)	305 calories
1 cup mashed potatoes (237 cals)	1 small baked sweet potato (54 cals)	183 calories
1 cup plain spaghetti (221 cals)	1 cup spaghetti squash (42 cals)	179 calories
2 slices Swiss cheese (213 cals)	1 Alouette Portions (40 cals)	173 calories
1 cup premium ice cream (266 cals)	1 Healthy Choice Greek Frozen Yogurt (100 cals)	166 calories
¼ cup pancake syrup (184 cals)	½ cup frozen blueberries, microwaved (40 cals)	144 calories
1 Reese's Big Cup peanut butter cup (200 cals)	2 Dove Promises Silky Smooth Peanut Butter Milk Chocolates (88 cals)	112 calories

Activate Your Anti-Aging Diet Now!

1   **Stay true to the 3-4-5 Plan** Losing weight is about as easy as it gets when you follow the simple 3-4-5 rule: 300 calories at breakfast, 400 calories at lunch, and 500 calories at dinner, with satisfying between-meals snacks.

2   **Be prepared for great eating** Stocking up on ingredients and grab-and-go foods will help you stick to the plan even when life gets in the way. Even those who aren't dieting can reap the health benefits of the meal and snack plan, so think about trying something new for the whole family.

3   **Take a pleasure trip to weight loss** The 7 Years Younger Meal Plan is a delicious journey. All the counting and planning have been done for you. All you have to do is decide which of our tasty meals you're going to try first.

For more expert diet anti-aging advice, get our free special report Eat to Look & Feel Younger *at 7yearsyounger.com/eattolookyoung.*

Chapter 3

Ready, Set…Let's Get Started

I't's time to erase a lot of what you've ever thought about dieting. The true sign of a successful diet is not that you've been able to lose weight; it's that you're able to keep it off.

The *7 Years Younger Anti-Aging Breakthrough Diet* is designed to give you seven full weeks of guided meal planning to ensure that you're burning more calories than you're taking in, but it's also about teaching you what you need to know about how to eat well for the rest of your life to keep managing your weight. In this chapter, we'll share diet-control strategies that science has proven will work. These are the tactics we consider to be the crème de la crème because they are designed not just to make you a weight-loss winner but to make it possible to *stay* a winner—forever.

On Your Mark

The diet starts Monday! Or maybe it's New Year's Day, or the day the kids go back to school, or the day after you get back from vacation. Whatever date you've decided to make Day One, you may know from past experience that just the anticipation of going on a diet can make people do things they ordinarily would never do—like take a serving spoon to a gallon of ice cream before the clock strikes midnight on the eve of D(iet) Day. It's a proven fact borne out by mountains of research and anecdotal evidence that the thought of going on a diet and the anticipated deprivation—*I'm going for it big-time tonight, because the diet starts tomorrow*—can trigger the mother of all binges. There's even a name for it: the Last Supper Effect. One way to think about it is to compare it to the way you feel after a big holiday meal. Too often, we stuff ourselves until we need to unbuckle our belts or unzip our pants, or we wind up on the couch groaning about how full we are.

We want to put your mind at ease right from the get-go, because you don't have to worry about deprivation on the 7 *Years Younger Anti-Aging Breakthrough Diet*. There is a variety of food for you to enjoy, so you won't be feeling hungry. There's no need to take yourself out for one last hurrah before this diet; this plan is designed to avoid giving you the feeling of deprivation that other diets create.

"I was pretty surprised to find that I can be satisfied eating healthy foods prepared with interesting herbs and spices and not at all crave fried or processed foods," says David Sigman. "I don't feel deprived at all, and feeling so much better is a bonus!" Our panelists started out on a Monday, nearly a week after we gathered them in *Good Housekeeping*'s New York City offices to introduce them to the diet. They spent their time getting prepared, just as you will want to. And, yes, many of them reported experiencing a Last Supper Effect. So, to set yourself up for success, get yourself in the right mindset with this 7 *Years Younger Anti-Aging Breakthrough Diet* kick start:

Make a contract with yourself Take a minute to think about the 7 Years Younger Diet Pledge you wrote at the beginning of the book. If you made that commitment, keeping those words in mind and in sight gives you a big mental edge in your ability to stick with the program. A Dominican University of California study that examined the success of goal-setters found that those who wrote down their aspirations were more likely to reach them than people who merely made mental vows. Photocopy your pledge and post it somewhere visible to inspire yourself—on your bathroom mirror, on the refrigerator, on your desktop or computer screen...wherever you can see it often. Your pledge is there as a reminder of your goals and priorities, as something you can refer to time and again to help keep yourself focused when temptation is getting the best of your willpower. Consider your pledge one of your most important tools for success.

Don't go it alone Give yourself a fair shot by teaming up with a buddy. Multiple studies, including a well-known joint investigation by Brown University Medical School and the University of Minnesota, have found that dieters who have a partner are more likely to stick with their regimens and lose more weight than those who go it alone. They also have less trouble keeping it off. The secret goes beyond commiserating over hunger pangs, swapping low-cal recipes, and working out together, though all of those things help. Diet buddies are mentally connected. Research shows that they truly support each other, offering encouragement when someone hits a rough patch and celebrating together when victories are achieved. A victory for one means a victory for both.

There were two couples among our test panelists, and both pairs felt that working together on their goal was a chief driver of their success. Daniel Chin admitted that at first he just went along with the diet to support his wife, Gean. But then he lost 12 pounds, and in the process he became a true convert to healthy eating—important, considering that he makes most of the family meals. Michele and Neil Fredman teamed up to

Michele Fredman

"Having a partner made it much easier to stick to the diet"

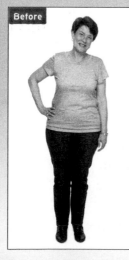

Before

Age
61

Height
5'4½"

Weight lost
7½ lbs.

Inches lost
6½ in.

90

STRUGGLES IN PAST DIETING HISTORY "I've dieted on other programs successfully, but I always regained the lost weight and a little more on top of that."

WHY 7YY "For its emphasis on improving my appearance and general health, and also to be happier about the way I look at our daughter's wedding. This plan is an easy-to-follow road map for eating, exercise, and skin care that is stunning in its simplicity and flexibility. In particular, it suggested meals and snacks that are tasty and nutritionally balanced. I'm losing weight pretty consistently, and I'm seeing that my fear of gaining wrinkles while losing pounds was essentially unfounded."

SUCCESS SECRET "I am now eating fruit, a Kind bar, and yogurt in various combinations for lunch and snacks and staying completely away from the cookies, candy, and general junk foods that people love to bring to share in our office. We are now buying only no-sugar-added ice cream. The most important thing is that we are now very mindful of portion sizes and the calories in processed foods. I can't say enough about the advantages of dieting with one's spouse."

PROUDEST OF "The amount of weight my husband, Neil, has lost— 23 pounds—and the fact that we have been able to stick with the diet." (See Neil Fredman on page 114.)

FAVORITE 7YY RECIPE "Curried Chicken Salad [page 252]."

BEST ADVICE FOR OTHER DIETERS "Going on the diet with a partner makes it much easier to do the shopping and removes the temptation of eating fattening foods that otherwise find their way into the kitchen when only one person in the household is dieting. Mind your portions, and eat enough of the planned menus to keep from getting too hungry."

Want to be a panelist for a future 7 Years Younger plan? Sign up at 7yearsyounger.com/panelist to be considered.

lose weight for their daughter's upcoming wedding and really cheered on each other's successes. "We'd each sit with the recipes and check off those we were interested in trying," says Michele, "and that's what we'd have for our dinners." Each beamed about being "so proud" of his or her spouse's results. "One morning Michele told me my clothes were hanging on me and I'd better find something smaller to wear," says Neil. "That felt really good to hear."

Anybody can be your diet buddy, but your best bet is usually someone in your family who will be eating off the same set of plates.

Prepare to journal Keeping a diet diary is the number one strategy for successful weight loss. One study, for example, tracked nearly 1,700 dieters who conscientiously wrote down everything they ate and drank in a food diary and calibrated the calories. They ended up losing twice as much weight as dieters who followed all the same dietary rules except for keeping a diary. And the more faithful they were about recording their meals each day, the more weight they lost.

When we launched our panelists on the 7 *Years Younger Anti-Aging Breakthrough Diet*, we gave them a notebook and asked them to record everything they ate, even though they had committed to following a seven-week meal plan. The majority kept track of every morsel faithfully. In fact, for many it was an eye-opener. "Keeping the diary showed me how much sugar I was eating throughout the day," says Elizabeth Worthy, 43, a publishing events manager. "I was drinking a lot of calories in sodas. Just giving that up probably played a key role in my losing 11 pounds in seven weeks."

Malaika Adero says keeping the food journal did more than help her achieve her 8-pound loss. "It teaches you so much about how much food you really eat," she says. "I found out that eating well means eating quality food in the right quantity."

Keeping a journal is important for more than just keeping track of

You Can Bet on It

Diet bets are popping up everywhere—online, in gyms, in weight-loss classes, and as informal wagers among friends, spouses, and coworkers. They're popular because they work: A multicenter study found that dieters who stood to lose money if they didn't succeed in shedding weight were about five times as likely to reach their goal as those with no financial stake in the outcome. Half of the gamblers dropped 16 pounds in 16 weeks—a congratulatory pound a week!—compared with just 10% of a group of non-bettors.

In a University of North Carolina at Chapel Hill study, the dieters who were told they'd pocket $14 for every 1% of lost body weight were nearly five and a half times more likely to shed 5% of their body weight than another group not offered a monetary incentive.

Putting money, ego, and bragging rights on the line is a potent formula for keeping up your motivation. "If eating chocolate cake tonight means you'll lose $10 or $50 at your next weigh-in, dessert suddenly isn't very attractive," says Dean Karlan, Ph.D., a Yale University behavioral economist. After losing 40 pounds in a personal bet with a friend, Karlan went on to found stickk.com, one of the first online weight-loss betting sites.

The big question is: Could this work for you? Researchers, diet veterans, and founders of betting websites say wagering could be your ticket to weight-loss success if:

- **You thrive on competition,** whether it's at sports, board games, making the best dish for the church potluck supper, or trying to improve on your own best results.

- **You know how to lose weight,** but you have trouble sticking to a diet. Betting can keep you motivated for the long haul.

- **You need a wake-up call.** You think you're following a good weight-loss program, but the scale isn't budging because you're letting yourself cheat or slack off on exercise.

calories. It also helps you keep in touch with your hunger cues. Use it to record your levels of hunger throughout the day, how you feel after a meal, and how you enjoyed the meal you just ate. It's also a place to keep tabs on your exercise progress and how it is affecting your energy level.

These days it is easier than ever to keep track of your diet progress. You can try our *7 Years Younger Anti-Aging Breakthrough Diet Workbook*. Or if you prefer, you can sign up for any one of the numerous diet diaries you can buy or get for free on your smartphone or computer—myfitnesspal.com and loseit.com are just two examples. Whichever option you choose, be sure to record what you've eaten as soon as you've swallowed your last bite. Memory can be selective, and it is very easy to lose track of an extra snack, or of having taken a handful of M&M's out of the bowl on a colleague's desk while you're chatting with her.

Purge your pantry and fridge See food, eat food. Studies by eating-behavior expert Brian Wansink, Ph.D., of Cornell University, confirm that we pop food into our mouths simply because it's there, regardless of whether we're hungry. It's just too easy to reach for fattening, and often unhealthy, items when they're staring back at us, so why tempt yourself? Empty your pantry and refrigerator of temptation, and you'll be doing yourself and your family a favor. Embarking on a healthy lifestyle means learning to eat better meals and snacks, and this doesn't just apply to dieters. Get rid of the white sugar and flour and fill your pantry with whole grains, especially in breakfast cereals. Replace white pasta with whole-grain varieties. Don't keep temptations such as ice cream and cupcakes on hand. Consider them a luxury in the truest sense and make them a special "let's-go-out-for [you fill in the treat]" event.

Go food shopping for the week Be prepared! Go over your meal options for Week 1 and decide on the meals you are going to eat. Make a list, then go food shopping. Our panelists reported that it took them longer to food-shop for the first week—for most of them, it hadn't been customary to

Never Go In Hungry

You might have heard it before, but it is important advice: Never go to the supermarket on an empty stomach; no matter how focused you try to be, you'll feel like a kid in a toy store. There's no reason to make things so hard on yourself! "I actually write out my grocery list in the order in which I encounter items in my supermarket," says Porscha Burke. "It helps me get in and out of the store quickly and avoid the cookie, candy, and cracker aisles."

Research shows that these tactics also work:

- **Arm yourself with a list, and stick to it.** Not only will this keep you from straying, but it will also keep you from spending too much.

- **If you have to squeeze in food shopping when your tank is a little low,** pick up a small snack when you get to the store—an energy bar, some string cheese, or another low-calorie snack—and eat it first. Just include the empty wrapper with your goods for checkout.

- **Go it alone.** Not only will it speed up your trip, but you'll also avoid the temptation to cave in to your kids' or spouse's demands.

Depending on where you live, you might be able to try this strategy: Place your grocery order online and have it delivered. Virtual shopping makes you stick to your list, a diet strategy proven to work. When researchers followed a group of virtual shoppers and compared them to dieters who shopped in the traditional way for eight weeks, the virtual shoppers ended up with fewer fattening products and less total food in their cupboards.

keep healthy staples on hand. But after that, food shopping did not take any longer than usual. So plan on having a big, ceremonial trip to the store for the first week; after that, you'll just want to shop for the foods on each week's meal plan. Or, for a helpful, step-by-step guide, pick up a copy of the 7 *Years Younger Anti-Aging Breakthrough Diet Workbook.*

Think small to get smaller However much weight you have to lose, don't focus on a long-term struggle. It can be really discouraging to think,

Argh, I have to lose 50 pounds. Or 60, or even just 20. Instead, think of it in terms of many incremental successes of five pounds.

Set mini goals for yourself, like making an effort to start eating vegetables at every meal or cooking dinner rather than getting takeout. These little achievements help lead to feelings of success and frame weight loss positively. After each success, celebrate, but not with food. Buy yourself a pair of earrings or tickets to a football game, or get a manicure—find rewards that make you happy in a non-food-related way, and celebrate small milestones to keep your momentum going.

Get a good night's sleep A study conducted at Stanford University found that people who routinely slept only five or six hours a night were 6 to 8 pounds heavier than those who got seven to eight hours of shut-eye. Another study at Eastern Virginia Medical School found that thin people, on average, get two hours more sleep a week than overweight people.

Missed zzz's can put you in a state of chronic fatigue, making you more likely to eat (usually carbs and sweet foods) to keep up your energy. Fatigue also plays tug-of-war with your willpower—something researchers at McLean Hospital in Belmont, MA, found out when they hooked up people with flagging eyelids in the middle of the day to functional-MRI machines and showed them photos of high-calorie goodies like chocolate cake. The MRI readings revealed lower activity in the area of the brain that regulates willpower in those tired people than in the well-rested.

A good night's sleep is also essential to looking good and feeling good. It's the time when your body performs most of its cellular repair, it helps your hormones maintain a healthy pattern, and it reboots your brain.

Get Set

These scientifically proven principles are basic diet tenets of the *7 Years Younger Anti-Aging Breakthrough Diet*. These strategies will help make following the diet all the easier.

Breakfast of champions Breakfast is the meal of weight-loss winners. Why? Because it wakes up your metabolism and gets it out of its nighttime slump. "Your metabolism slows while you sleep, and the process of digesting food in the morning revs it up," says Christine Gerbstadt, M.D., a spokesperson for the American Dietetic Association. Research shows that breakfast eaters typically consume about 100 fewer calories per day—that adds up to 10 pounds a year!—and weigh less than breakfast skippers. And when experts from the University of Colorado Health Sciences Center surveyed more than 3,000 successful dieters who had lost 30 pounds or more and kept it off for at least a year, they found that eating breakfast was the one commonality they all shared.

The reason? "People who skip breakfast are more likely to snack impulsively during the morning," says Joan Salge Blake, R.D., clinical associate professor at Boston University's Sargeant College of Health & Rehabilitation Sciences. That makes you susceptible to whatever's close by, like the donuts at your staff meeting.

For many breakfast skippers, running out the door on empty has nothing to do with some heroic diet ploy. They simply aren't hungry. However, the "eat breakfast" dictum does not mean you have to shovel it in the moment you get out of bed. The sooner you eat after waking up, the better, but as long as you eat within three hours of getting out of bed, you'll still reap the metabolic benefit.

"I never ate breakfast before going on the 7 *Years Younger Anti-Aging Breakthrough Diet*, and I still can't eat as soon as I get up," says panelist Leigh Gillam. "Now, faithfully at 10 A.M., I heat up some oatmeal, and it keeps me satisfied. When lunchtime comes around, I'm not hungry like I used to be."

Don't skip any meals A study conducted at Virginia Commonwealth University found that dieters were able to lose impressive amounts of weight—23 pounds over four months, and another 17 pounds over the next four months—simply because they didn't bypass meals.

Skipping meals is a weight-loss strategy that's sure to backfire. (Your own diet history may even remind you of that fact.) Our biology just isn't designed to let us go without food for long stretches. When you fast or skip meals, it's a pretty sure bet that at some point you're "suddenly" going to feel famished. With your willpower on the edge, you're liable to eat something you'll regret.

Become a label reader Here's a secret you might not know: Thin people tend to check food labels. A recent international study tracked the food-shopping habits of 25,640 Americans and found that women who read nutritional labels when food shopping weigh nearly 9 pounds less than women who do not. The study also found that women are better label readers than men: 74% of women, versus only 58% of men, look at nutritional information.

Dieter's Top Tip

Be Prepared to Eat

Melissa Berman kicked off her *7 Years Younger Anti-Aging Breakthrough Diet* experience by making her breakfasts, lunches, and snacks in the morning or even the night before so they would be there when she was hungry. "For me, planning ahead was key to sticking with it," she says. "When I was hungry, the meal or snack was already there. It kept me from heading for the first convenience food I could get my hands on, such as a bagel, which was my custom in the past." It also helped make her one of the 7 Years Younger champion losers, at 19 pounds and 6 1/2 inches shed in just seven weeks.

Breakfast on the Run

For people who can't face food when they first wake up, a bar can be a good on-the-go fast-breaker an hour or two into the day. The problem is, many of them are little more than fancy candy bars.

That's why the Good Housekeeping Research Institute's Nutrition Lab set out to find the breakfast bars that best matched the nutritional and calorie goals of the 3-4-5 Plan. For our test, volunteers nibbled their way through 28 nationally available varieties to come up with six winners. Although these are the best of the best, some still contain more sugar than we'd like; that's why you won't see most of these bars in our meal plan. However, when you're in a bind, any of them will do! To make a bar *7 Years Younger Anti-Aging Breakthrough Diet*-friendly, have it with a piece of fruit or a 12-ounce nonfat latte.

Breakfast Bars

Our requirements: At least 170 calories, 6 grams of protein, and 3 grams of fiber, and no more than 3 grams of saturated fat. And the winners are:

- **Clif Bar White Chocolate Macadamia Nut** *(250 calories)* The chewy texture pleased our panelists.

- **Kind Nuts & Spices in Madagascar Vanilla Almond** *(210 calories)* Our testers loved the "natural-tasting" bar with "lots of nuts."

- **Luna Nutz Over Chocolate** *(180 calories)* Overall, this chocolate-dipped bar was a winner.

- **Luna Peanut Honey Pretzel** *(190 calories)* The "sweet and salty combination" and the "peanut butter flavor" proved irresistible.

- **Rickland Orchards Toasted Coconut Greek Yogurt Bar** *(170 calories)* The chocolate flavor was a hit, though the yogurt coating got mixed reviews.

- **ThinkThin Caramel Chocolate Dipped Mixed Nuts Crunch Bar** *(190 calories)* "A good combination of chocolate and nuts," said most testers.

Another study found that most people have a short attention span when it comes to reading nutrition labels. Although most consumers did view labels, very few viewed every component on any label, report Dan J. Graham, Ph.D., and Robert W. Jeffrey, Ph.D., who conducted the research at the University of Minnesota School of Public Health. Reading nutrition facts labels is key to staying true to your diet. Make sure you check a product's serving size in addition to the calories. Looks can be deceiving: What might look to you like one serving can actually be two or even more. Pay attention to the saturated fat, protein, fiber, and sugar content. As a rule of thumb, remember this: The higher, the better for fiber and protein, and the lower, the better for sugars and saturated fat.

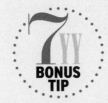

How to Spot Trans Fat

Just because a label says "trans-fat free" does not mean the item actually is. Because of a labeling loophole, products can still contain small amounts of the dangerous man-made fat without saying so! Manufacturers can claim a product is "trans-fat free" as long as its trans-fat content is under half a gram per serving, not per package.

Trans fats have been linked to increases in the risk of heart disease and obesity and may be associated with an increased risk of certain forms of cancer. The Food and Drug Administration and the American Heart Association have declared that there is "no safe level for human consumption" of them. To spy trans fats still hiding in food, look for the term "hydrogenated" or "partially hydrogenated" on the ingredient list; either is an indicator that trans fats reside inside.

Check your portion sizes The saying "Everything in moderation" is particularly true when it comes to portion size. It's easy to overestimate the size of one cup or three ounces, especially when you're just getting started. Sales associate Jeanne Fishwick, 53, learned this when she stopped counting the chips she was eating for her snack because she thought she could "eyeball it." "I gained weight back that week," she says. "When I suspected that the chips might be a problem, I went back to counting them. That got me back on track." She went on to lose 8 pounds in seven weeks.

The 7 *Years Younger Anti-Aging Breakthrough Diet* recipes and meal plan are carefully proportioned to give you an exact number of calories and nutrients throughout your day. Using our recipes and following the meal plan will help you learn to intuitively estimate what a portion size should be when you're dining out and when you're preparing your own recipes.

As a rough estimate, here is a reminder of what a portion size looks like:

- 3 ounces of fish, poultry, or meat = a smartphone
- An ounce of cheese = four dice
- 2 tablespoons of dressing = a shot glass
- A half cup of grains, rice, or pasta = a tennis ball
- A small dinner roll = a computer mouse
- A quarter-cup of nuts = a large egg
- A teaspoon of butter = a Scrabble tile

Resign from the clean-plate club We're all getting a little bit bigger because we are eating large portions in restaurants and dishing out larger portions at home. And we tend to eat until the plate is clean, no matter what.

Cornell University behavior expert Brian Wansink proved the point in a novel experiment in which he gave "bottomless bowls" of soup—the bowls automatically kept refilling—to an unknowing group of volunteers and gave regular bowls of soup to others. Those eating from the never-ending bowls wound up consuming 73% more soup than the others before they were told to stop. When asked if they were full, a common reply was, "How can I be full? I still have half a bowl left!"

So pay attention to your satiety cues, not how much is still on the plate or in the bowl. That's one reason why it's important to eat slowly: It takes about 20 minutes for your brain to register what you've eaten and tell you when you've had enough to eat. You should only eat until you're comfortably full, not stuffed. It means still feeling energetic after a meal, not sluggish. This requires putting down your fork before you feel uncomfortable. Eat slowly, and pay attention to what your stomach is saying.

It Pays to Measure

Measuring is a calorie-saver that catches many people by surprise. Just how far astray can you go when you freely pour what you think is about a teaspoon of sugar or a tablespoon of olive oil? That's what we wanted to find out, so we had our nutrition lab ask a group of volunteers to prep a few meals and snacks following our intentionally vague instructions about amounts. No surprise: They came up with vastly different interpretations of portions. Imagine what these results can do to a diet:

Testers were told to	Lightest hand	Heaviest hand	Calorie difference
"Pour some dressing over the salad"	1/8 Tbsp. (9 cals)	2 1/3 Tbsp. (169 cals)	160
"Grab a handful of nuts"	6 almonds (41 cals)	30 almonds (207 cals)	166
"Put a schmear of peanut butter on a slice of bread"	2/3 tsp. (19 cals)	1 1/2 Tbsp. (141 cals)	122
"Drizzle olive oil in a pan" (to sauté broccoli)	2/3 tsp. (26 cals)	1 3/4 Tbsp. (209 cals)	183

Downsize your dining ware The key to eating less is serving yourself less, and the best way to do so, suggests Wansink, is to use smaller tableware. The size of plates and bowls has been gradually increasing over the generations; in fact, the average dinner plate has grown in size 22% over the last century. "This increase in plate size approximately mirrors the increase in portion size and in the availability and affordability of food," says Wansink, adding that we have become increasingly less able to accurately estimate how many calories we eat as portion sizes expand.

The idea of "large" is just a trap to make us eat more. For example, Wansink's experiments found that:

- When 30 students were given different-size bowls of Chex Mix to munch on at a Super Bowl party, those eating out of 16-cup bowls ate 53% more than those eating out of bowls that fit about eight cups.

- When 98 adults were asked to prepare a spaghetti dinner for two, those given a half-full 32-ounce box to cook from prepared 29% more than those given a full 16-ounce box.

- When 161 moviegoers were given popcorn, those munching from

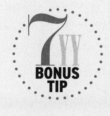

Forgo "Family-Style" Dining

Plating food in the kitchen rather than bringing it to the table family-style is a strategy that helped women eat 10% fewer calories, reports a Cornell experiment. You also want to plate food in the right proportions, something that will become second nature as you start making the *7 Years Younger Anti-Aging Breakthrough Diet* recipes. The *Good Housekeeping* rule of thumb: One-quarter of your meal should be protein, half should be fruits and vegetables, and a quarter should be grains.

eight-ounce buckets ate 53% more than those who had four-ounce buckets. Even moviegoers given stale, two-week-old popcorn managed to eat 34% more popcorn when they were given larger buckets!

Train yourself to respond to internal cues The environment in which we dine can influence how much we eat. Wansink demonstrated this in an experiment in which he asked 133 Parisians and 145 Chicagoans how they determined when they were finished eating dinner. The leading replies from Paris: People stopped when they "were no longer hungry" or when the meal "no longer tasted good"—what Wansink described as internal cues of satiety. The leading replies from Chicago: "When my plate's empty" or when a TV show was over—external cues. However, no matter where they lived, overweight people relied on different cues than normal-weight people. "They relied more on external cues," said Wansink.

Getting in touch with your internal cues is largely a matter of turning off the external buzz. Keep meals away from television, smartphones, homework, and music. Everything you eat, even if it is just a snack, should be eaten without distractions.

The same goes for eating while you work. "Your desk is a minefield of distractions, so chances are you'll be multitasking while eating," warns Elisa Zied, M.S., R.D., author of *Nutrition at Your Fingertips*. "This can leave you not only unsatisfied, but also likely to eat past fullness." Remember, the best meals are the ones that get your undivided attention. If work is front and center, then enjoying a good lunch is not. If you must dine at your desk, be sure to stop working, put your computer to sleep and your smartphone in a drawer, and concentrate on eating.

Go for the Win

There's an old joke in which a visitor stops a maestro on the street and asks how to get to Carnegie Hall. The answer: "Practice, practice, practice."

That's our advice, too, for establishing healthy eating habits. Practice these healthy strategies often, and they eventually will become second nature.

Eat your veggies first Evidence suggests that if you eat the lower-calorie items on your plate first, it will help take the edge off your hunger and you'll be less likely to overeat. With the recipes and menus on the 7 *Years Younger Anti-Aging Breakthrough Diet*, you have the opportunity to savor low-calorie foods at every meal, so take advantage of it!

Keep food out of sight Yes, out of sight *is* out of mind. A simple experiment by Cornell researchers showed how easy it is to mindlessly eat. Observing the snacking habits of people who kept candy on their desks at work, the researchers found that snackers had a tendency to reach for M&M's more often when they were displayed in a clear jar than when they were kept in an opaque container. If you can't get food out of sight, at least put it in a container you can't see through.

Eat for satiety, not fullness In the Okinawan islands of Japan, where some of the world's longest-lived people reside and few are overweight, it is common to practice "hara hachi bu" at every meal. Loosely translated, it means "Eat until you're 80% full," says Bradley J. Willcox, M.D., a

Dieter's Top Tip

Keep Healthy Choices
◀ at Eye Level

"Eating the 7 Years Younger way has become my new way of life," says Elizabeth Worthy, who lost 11 pounds in seven weeks. "If you're not seeing bad food choices when you open the refrigerator, you won't be eating or preparing them." The biggest change that led to her success: "Stocking my refrigerator with healthy choices that stare back at me when I open it."

Hawaii-based expert in geriatric medicine who studied and wrote a book about Okinawan longevity. The islanders aren't walking around hungry, explains Dr. Wilcox; they just know to stop before they have to loosen their belts. It's cultural wisdom that's right on target.

To help make the practice of eating for satiety a habit, consciously rate your hunger on a scale of 1 to 10 at every meal, with 1 being "famished" and 10 "letting your belt out to make room for what you just ate." Try beginning each meal the way the Okinawans do—or make up your own mantra to remind yourself to eat mindfully. Notice the clock and try to make your meal last at least 20 minutes. When you are halfway through your meal, put your fork down, rest a few minutes, and rate your fullness level. Eat another few bites and stop again. When your rating gets to a 7, see if you can push your plate away. If you can, good for you! When you get to 8, stop no matter what. If you're still hungry after your first helping, get up and do something for five or 10 minutes: Pay some bills, fold laundry, or read a section of the paper. This little exercise helps you identify the difference between actual hunger and eating out of habit. If after 10 minutes you're still not feeling satiated, then it's OK to come back for more; in most instances, though, your hunger will have subsided.

Eat s-l-o-w-l-y and with purpose When you have lunch with a thin friend, who usually finishes first? Often, wolfing down food can be one of the big reasons for a weight problem. Research into the psychology of problem eaters shows that mindless munching leads to overindulgence. In our full-speed-ahead society, we're rarely just sitting down to enjoy a meal; usually we're multitasking by watching television, reading the newspaper, playing Words With Friends, talking business over lunch, or doing any number of other activities that keep us from really paying attention to how our body is responding to what we're eating.

To mentally connect to food in a healthy way, consciously pay attention to what you are eating: Eat slowly, pause between bites, and enjoy the

Ask the EXPERT

Samantha B. Cassetty, M.S., R.D.
Nutrition Director, GHRI

Q *I have a real sweet tooth and love all things sugary. Any tips for staying on track?*

Samantha says: I have one, too, but I also have a few tricks that help me control my cravings rather than letting them control me. Cutting back on sugar, which we've done in the 7 Years Younger Meal Plan, is a good place to start. (The healthy limit: Six teaspoons of added sugar a day.) It will feel tough at first, but after a few days, your taste buds will adjust—I promise!

Having a planned indulgence is another great strategy. You'll find treats like dessert-worthy Chobani Bites yogurt, squares of dark chocolate, and no-added-sugar ice creams and puddings built into your menu, so you won't feel deprived.

Finally, I suggest practicing the mindful-eating techniques outlined on pages 106–111 while having dessert. These tips help me savor my sweets (rather than wolf them down), and they'll be useful whether you're enjoying an everyday treat (like those mentioned above) or a more rare and indulgent one.

Q *When I'm at the supermarket, what low-cal/low-fat salad dressings should I look for?*

Samantha says: For oil-based dressings, my general rule is to look for versions that have about 45 calories per two-tablespoon serving. Don't worry about the fat. For that number of calories, you won't get much, and the fat in salad dressing tends to be a healthy variety like olive, canola, or soybean oil. Plus, the fat helps you absorb the stay-young nutrients, like beta-carotene, that the veggies provide. Sugar can add up, though, so make sure the dressing you choose has no more than 4 grams (that's one teaspoon per two-tablespoon serving). Newman's Own Lite Balsamic is my go-to bottled vinaigrette; it meets all of these parameters. Love creamy dressings like ranch? Light versions have more calories than vinaigrette— about 80 per two-tablespoon portion. GHRI testers rated Marzetti Light Classic Ranch tops in the category.

Melissa Berman

"I ate just because food was there, not because I was hungry"

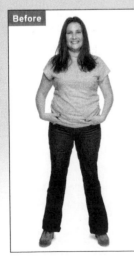

Before

Age
46

Height
5' 4"

Weight lost
19 lbs.

Inches lost
6½ in.

STRUGGLES IN PAST DIETING HISTORY Melissa had never been on a diet before this one. But, says the stay-at-home mom from New York City, "I wasn't blessed with skinny genes, and as I discovered, it gets a lot easier to put on weight as you grow older. At age 46, I didn't like where I was headed."

The on-the-go mother of two young boys blames her 40-pound weight gain over the years on falling into bad food habits. "I'd put food in my mouth when I was making the kids' breakfasts and packing their lunches," she says. "At dinner, I'd finish what they didn't eat. I got into the junk food habit. I'd eat just because the food was there, not because I was hungry."

WHY 7YY "It includes a large variety of foods, even chocolate, and you get to eat a lot of healthy carbohydrates."

SUCCESS SECRET "Paying attention to every bite I put in my mouth. I've found food tastes better when I only eat when I'm hungry."

PROUDEST OF "Losing my 'baby fat.' My babies are now 9 and 11."

FAVORITE 7YY RECIPES "I loved so many, but Strawberry Cereal [page 222] for breakfast, Spinach & Nectarine Salad [page 240] for lunch, and Pomegranate-Glazed Salmon [page 271] for dinner, just to name a few."

BEST ADVICE FOR OTHER DIETERS "Food-shop for the week ahead, make and pack your meals and snacks the night before or in the morning, and carry a water bottle with you. When you get hungry, you'll already have the healthy choice with you and won't be grabbing junk or making the wrong food choice."

flavor. Notice the texture, the temperature, the aroma. Is it sweet or savory? Juicy or crunchy? Can you detect a note of spice?

When you eat slowly, you not only appreciate the taste of your food, but also take longer to eat it, which gives your brain the 20 minutes it needs to signal your stomach that you've had enough. And it works: In one study, women who took half an hour to eat a pasta lunch consumed almost 70 fewer calories than those who scarfed their lunch down in nine minutes. Save that many calories at two meals a day for a year, and you could lose nearly 15 pounds!

Make every bite count Even when you prepare your own meal or order a healthful option at a restaurant, you can't control whether your dining companion is going to follow suit. And when a giant unhealthy dish shows up at the table, it's tempting to ask for a bite or to accept an offer to try just a little! Sounds harmless enough, but weight-loss experts say no: Whether you're nabbing french fries off of your child's plate or sampling your way through making dinner, each bite adds, on average, an extra 25 calories to your day. That means that regularly grazing on the

Dieter's Top Tip

Develop "Selective Willpower"

Neil Fredman admits he'd always been an all-or-nothing kind of guy when it comes to food. "It wasn't one cookie; it was the whole bag," he says. But the *7 Years Younger Anti-Aging Breakthrough Diet* turned him on to a new strategy. "I now make evaluations about the foods I want to eat," he says. "I look at it as a cost/benefit. For example, if the cookie I want to eat is 100 calories, I ask myself if it's worth the calories. If the answer is no, I simply pass on it." It's selective willpower, and it works—in Neil's case, to the tune of 23 pounds in seven weeks.

food that's around you rather than sticking to what's on your plate three or four times a day can add up to an extra 7½ pounds a year. When researchers from the University of North Carolina at Chapel Hill looked at more than 30 years of American-style eating patterns, they identified between-meals munchies as the number one reason for the rise in our calorie intake. Snacking now accounts for 25% of all calories consumed by Americans, averaging about 580 calories a day. That hardly fits the definition of a snack!

It's important to be mindful of the impact that even a casual nibble here and there can have on your ability to achieve your weight-management goals; that doesn't mean you can't ever nibble, but you should factor it into your meal planning if you want to stay on track.

Follow the command "Sit!" You expect your dog to follow the rules at treat time, and so should you. "It sounds so simple, but if you're going to eat, commit to sit," says Susan Albers, Psy.D., a psychologist at the Cleveland Clinic and author of *50 Ways to Soothe Yourself Without Food*. Eating only when you are seated allows you to appreciate what you are chewing, so you consume less instead of wolfing down your food. Think of all the occasions when we eat standing up—grabbing a freebie taste while pushing the supermarket cart down the aisle, reaching into the cookie jar while cleaning up the kitchen after dinner, sliding an hors d'oeuvre off the tray while in deep conversation at a cocktail party. They are all land mines of mindless eating.

Try something new at least once a week There are many factors behind a weight problem, and eating the wrong kinds of foods is high on the list. For most people, losing weight and changing their eating habits means needing to replace calorie- and fat-laden foods with new ones. Make it a habit to pick up something new in the produce section every time you food-shop, and give it a try. More than likely, you'll be discovering a new 7YY-friendly food.

Many people think they don't like certain vegetables, perhaps as a result of a bad experience—*Aunt Helen cooked string beans to death!* But when was the last time you tasted an asparagus stalk plucked fresh from the garden...or one of the relatively new fresh foods, such as Broccolini...or farro or quinoa? Swap vegetables for meat just once a week, and you could drop four pounds in a year without changing anything else. When Johns Hopkins researchers fed 54 men and women similar lunches—one mushroom-based, the other meat-based—the mushroom eaters consumed roughly 30 fewer grams of fat than the meat eaters. They also reported that eating the vegetable-based meal was just as satisfying as eating meat.

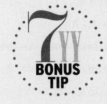

Practice Saying, "Later"

When faced with a diet-derailing temptation, don't give in or deprive yourself totally. Just tell yourself you're going to wait a little while. Simply **postponing the indulgence is the best way to curb your appetite,** say researchers from Portugal. To prove their theory, the researchers had 100 volunteers watch a movie with a bowl of candy in front of them. Some were told to eat freely, others were instructed not to touch, and a third group was advised they could have the sweets—but later on. When everyone was given the cue to dig in, the postponers ate the least—about half as much as those who had been told the treat was a no-no.

The reason is purely psychological. Telling yourself you can indulge at an unspecified future time subdues the craving in the moment, says researcher Nichole Mead, Ph.D., while having to "just say no" brings out your inner rebel.

It was unanimous: The part of the diet our panel of dieters loved the most was trying out new recipes. It offered a venture into something new every day—the ultimate real incentive to stay on the road to success.

Brown-bag it Avoid the unknown calories that may be lurking in your workplace cafeteria or at popular lunchtime eateries by brown-bagging the take-along lunch items offered in the 7 Years Younger Meal Plan and in our recipe section. Researchers at the Fred Hutchinson Cancer Research Center found that women who packed their own lunches lost five more pounds during a year of dieting than those who dined out for lunch weekly.

Switch to water We've talked about the health and beauty benefits of water, but drinking plenty of it can also be a great way to keep from eating too much. When Stanford researchers analyzed the diets of 173 overweight women, they found that those who consumed six glasses of water a day took in 200 fewer calories than people who shortchanged themselves on water. Another study found that people who drank two glasses of water before meals lost 41% more weight than those who didn't. Researchers theorize this is most likely due to the mind's interpreting a midday hunger pang as a need for food when what the body really needs is water. When panelist Gean Chin felt hungry between meals, she drank a big glass of water with lemon. "It really works to squelch hunger pangs," she says. Gean lost 6½ pounds and trimmed back 6 inches in seven weeks, proving that it's a winning strategy.

So when you feel that pang of hunger, have some water, wait five minutes, and see how you feel. If what you felt was thirst, the empty-stomach feeling will have gone away.

Shake a fist for willpower Here's a simple flexing exercise that saves calories: When you're deciding what to eat or whether you want more, boost your resolve by clenching your fist. Firming your muscles shores up your willpower, helping you overcome temptation, say University of Chicago researchers. They found this out through an experiment in which

Neil Fredman

"Constant feedback was the key to my success"

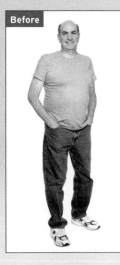

Before

Age
62

Height
6'3½"

Weight lost
23 lbs.

Inches lost
5½ in.

114

STRUGGLES IN PAST DIETING HISTORY "I was the quintessential yo-yo dieter. Every time I'd lose, I'd gradually drift back to bad eating habits."

WHY 7YY "I want to look my best at my daughter's wedding. I wanted a healthy diet to get me there."

SUCCESS SECRET "I like constant feedback, so I was diligent about counting calories and recording everything I'd eat. More specifically, weighing (no pun intended) the pros and cons before eating a specific thing, such as, *Are those chips worth 100 calories, or can I just skip them or eat something else?*"

PROUDEST OF "Doing this with my wife, Michele, and our both being successful at continuing toward our goals." (See Michele Fredman on page 90.)

FAVORITE 7YY RECIPE "Pulled Pork on a Bun [page 260]."

BEST ADVICE FOR OTHER DIETERS "Weigh yourself daily and record it in your diet journal. The feedback, either up or down, is helpful. Then you have to be prepared to follow the 'advice' that the scale is giving you, such as, 'You gained a pound yesterday; time to recalculate' or 'You lost a half-pound; keep up the good work.' In other words, success breeds success."

they passed out pens to a group of health-minded students, then directed them to hold on to the pen either tightly or loosely while ordering from the campus snack bar. Those who stiffened their grip reported feeling more in control of their decision and were more likely to choose fruit, tea, or yogurt instead of ice cream, croissants, or candy than the students who held on lightly. So make a fist at the buffet, and then move on.

Weigh yourself often Hop on the scale the morning you start the diet and frequently thereafter. It doesn't have to be daily, but it should be no less than once a week. More, though, is better. The reason for doing this is not to drive yourself crazy looking for little weight changes, but to give yourself frequent reminders that you're working toward a goal. Don't be alarmed if you're down a pound one day and up a pound or even two or three the next; fluctuations of one to three pounds are normal because of the retention of fluids.

Recalculate You're not going to be perfect. Slip-ups happen, and that's OK. What's important when they do is being mindful of the fact that you did slip up and empowering yourself to get back on track. It happens to everyone, and it happened to all our panelists. So what if you ate the whole thing? It doesn't mean you've failed. Even if it feels like you've blown your diet royally by eating everything you could poke your fork into at the buffet table, let go of your guilt, forgive yourself, and get back on board immediately.

Don't give up or binge-eat for the rest of the day and let a 600-calorie slip turn into a 6,000-calorie mistake. Instead, tell yourself to reset, just like the GPS in your car does when you take a wrong turn. You wouldn't continue driving in the wrong direction just because you turned left when you should have taken a right. Why would you continue along the wrong path on your diet? "Recalculate" was probably the word repeated most by our panelists when they communicated with one another on Facebook. And they are the proof that it works!

Activate Your Anti-Aging Diet Now!

1 **Prepare yourself for the start** Give yourself a few days to gear up for your diet. Arm yourself with a food diary—your primary tool for success. Get rid of diet temptations in your pantry and refrigerator and restock the shelves with healthy items that will make it easy to stay healthy even when you're on the go.

2 **Adopt healthy dieting principles** At the top of the list: Eat breakfast, never skip meals, and remember to balance your plate with an assortment of nutritious offerings. And never go more than three hours without food!

3 **Practice mindful eating** Before mealtime, take a minute to really consider what you're putting on your plate and why. Be thoughtful about how you balance your food. Eat without distractions, and be sure to savor every bite so you get the most out of it and don't accidentally eat past the point of fullness.

Now, as you start your anti-aging diet, is a great time to get even more expert advice and ongoing support. Sign up for our free weekly e-newsletter, Your Anti-Aging Tip Sheet, at 7yearsyounger.com/newsletter, and join us at facebook.com/7yearsyounger.

Chapter 4

Mind Over Platter

R esearch shows that thin people simply don't think about food the same way as the rest of us do. They don't start thinking about what they're going to eat the moment they make a dinner reservation or change their minds four times even before they step through the restaurant door. They don't try to starve themselves all day in preparation for food extravaganzas like a wedding, annual barbecue, fund-raiser, etc. They don't stick a fork in everybody else's desserts for "just a taste" at a dinner party.

People who tend to be career dieters are preoccupied with food, says Deborah Beck Bussis, L.S.W., who helps the overweight adopt healthy attitudes about food at the Beck Institute for Cognitive Therapy in sub-urban Philadelphia. They've got food on the brain, and they even tend to put labels on it that reflect their skewed thinking. There are "good"

Get in Touch With Your Dieting Style

Weight-loss expert Geneen Roth says there are two types of diet "personalities" that control the way we respond to food and our struggle to lose unwanted pounds. She calls people with these mindsets Restrictors and Permitters.

Restrictors are hypervigilant about food. They do well on diets—at least for a while. They find rules, tips, and lists comforting. They can tell you off the top of their head how many calories are in an apple, a baked potato, or a Subway turkey sub. "Restrictors like regulations because they provide a sense of control over uncertainty and unpredictability," says Roth, who is the author of several best-selling books including *Women, Food, and God*. Eventually, however, the deprivation becomes too much, and the Restrictor becomes intolerant of the rules. That's when the bingeing sets in. Restrictors then see their diets as ruined, but know that something else will come around another day. It becomes the perpetual yo-yo scenario.

Permitters are in denial about their weight. They hate rules and find them oppressive and suffocating. Even though they know they could stand to lose a few pounds (or more), they have a negative reaction to diet programs and food lists. "Permitters are the type of emotional eaters who say, 'Gee, I can't understand how I gained 10 pounds in the past two months. I thought I was

foods—the healthy items they know they should eat but don't want to—and "bad" foods, the foods they'd rather eat.

This doesn't mean you're destined to be a doomed dieter if you love food and love to eat. It's just that you might need a mindset adjustment to help maintain your weight loss once you reach your goal. "Without having a healthy attitude toward food, your chance of gaining back some, if not all, of the weight you lose is 96%," says Bussis. "Anybody who is motivated can make short-term behavioral changes, but if you struggle with weight loss, making long-term change means you have to alter the brain."

Mindset is a more important driver of weight-loss success than even doing well,'" says Roth. They suffer in secret over their weight and just don't know what to do about it because they feel dieting is hopeless.

Knowing your diet personality helps break the emotional cycle that inhibits weight loss. "It gives people tremendous relief to be able to recognize themselves as either Restrictors or Permitters," says Roth. "They become more aware of their needs and how to meet them, which helps them to begin the process of breaking free from their compulsive eating."

Both types of people can win at weight loss, says Roth. By recognizing your mindset, you can avoid the mental obstacles that could come between you and success. If you're a Permitter, you know you're going to struggle on a diet and break the rules. "So forget rules, and begin with awareness," says Roth. "Since Permitters use food to numb themselves and thus block out body signals, begin by paying attention to concrete physical sensations like hunger and fullness. Allow yourself to notice the plate of food in front of you and your body's response to it." She warns Permitters about giving themselves rigid rules: "Eat according to your physical hunger, and stop when you've had enough." For a Restrictor, "part of breaking away from compulsive eating is trusting that your body wants to feel well, to be nourished, and to thrive, and that if you listen to it, it won't betray you," says Roth.

the best meal plan can ever be. "Anyone can lose weight, but one reason people gain it back is because they haven't changed the mental habits that caused them to become overweight in the first place," says Bussis. Without making those changes, it's easier to slip back into old eating habits and routines that led to an unhealthy weight to begin with.

The mind is a powerful thing. It drives who we are and what we become, including our being thin or fat. And it works subtly. Research conducted at Yale University reveals just one example of how the mind drives the response to food. Scientists found that people who drank a milkshake they perceived as caloric (620 calories) declared that they felt fuller than when they unknowingly sipped the exact same shake, this time presented to them as low-calorie (140 calories). "Their satiety was consistent with what they believed they were consuming rather than the actual nutritional value of what they consumed," said Alia J. Crum, Ph.D., the lead researcher. And it had nothing to do with being in a dieting frame of mind: The people in the experiment were not on a diet!

Here's another example of how your mind controls what your stomach desires. When people were offered candy cut in half, they ate 60 fewer calories than people eating full-size pieces and reported being just as satisfied, a study in the *Journal of the American Dietetic Association* found. The reason? Their brains registered two pieces as a larger treat than a single one.

Winning at losing weight means getting control over a mindset that leads to overindulgence. Nowhere is this more obvious than at the Beck

Dieter's Top Tip

Her "Aha" Moment

Leigh Gillam is a gym junkie—and proof that you can be in good shape *and* be overweight. At 5' 7", she weighed 203 pounds despite devoting nearly two hours three times a week to vigorous exercise.

Her "aha" moment came when she realized her stops at a fast-food joint after the gym were sabotaging her effort to slim down. "I was telling myself I deserved to eat anything I wanted as a reward for working out so hard," she says. Gillam now has a new way of thinking about the rewards she wants to reap from her time at the gym: "Working out is hard and takes a lot of time. I decided I didn't want to waste it." She went cold turkey on junk food and turned to healthy eating. In seven weeks, she dropped 12 pounds and whittled an impressive 5 inches from her waist.

Institute, where counselors use cognitive therapy to help overweight people overcome the thought processes, both conscious and unconscious, that make them overeat. "We're not about the diet," says Bussis (the daughter of Judith Beck, Ph.D., the institute's director and author of *The Beck Diet*

Know Your Appetite Cues

Do you know the difference between hunger, desire, and cravings? Most dieters have difficulty distinguishing among the three, says the Beck Institute's Deborah Beck Bussis.

Hunger is the sensation you experience when you haven't eaten for hours and your stomach feels empty. It may even be talking back to you. **Desire** is the feeling that compels you to keep eating, even if you are full—like when you order cheesecake after eating a big steak dinner. A **craving** is a strong urge to eat—to the point where you have uncomfortable yearning and your body even tenses up.

There is only one cue that should lead you to eat: true hunger.

"A craving or desire is like an itch," says Bussis. "The more we pay attention to it, the worse it gets. On the other hand, if you get distracted, it will go away." When the urge to eat hits and you're not feeling real hunger, do something to get your mind off it—take a walk, call a friend, find something to organize, do whatever will get your mind off food.

Eating isn't meant to be automatic, though it sometimes feels like it: You see a brownie, you eat the brownie. However, that brownie crosses your lips because a voice in your head is saying, *So what if you aren't hungry? It looks good, so go for it.* Cognitive therapy works by challenging thought processes like this that lead to mindless eating, then training the brain to mute the voice of what the Beck Institute calls "sabotage thinking."

It's important to think about the difference between physical hunger and emotional hunger. You won't resolve emotional hunger with food; you need to figure out the real culprit—whether it's boredom, stress, sadness, or something else—and attack the problem with an appropriate solution, just as you provide your body with food when you're hungry.

Solution). "We're about making the diet work." And that means training the brain to think more like a thin person's.

It's easy to get stuck in the mindset of overeating. Researchers led by Cornell researcher Brian Wansink tested this by hosting a Super Bowl party for 50 students at an area bar that advertised unlimited chicken wings. At half the tables, waiters were instructed to continually scoop away the bones as the wings were eaten and deposit fresh wings. At the other tables, the bones piled up as waiters delivered more wings. In the end, the students faced with the discarded bones ended up eating 34% less than the students who had no visual record of how much they were eating. The students who ate the most also had a hard time believing how much they had consumed when they were shown the results at the end.

Yo-yo dieters and people who never achieve their weight-loss goal don't keep track of the "bones." They ignore their minds' cues and often eat way past fullness. Remember the goal from Chapter 3 of eating until you're 80% full? That's what you should be aiming for: being not stuffed, but comfortably full and satisfied.

Silence Your Mental Saboteurs

Sabotage thinking is what makes you go for seconds even when you're not actually hungry. It's eating just because the food is there, or because a friend says, "Let's share a dessert" after you've just announced you're full. It's what makes you dig into your mother-in-law's mega-calorie turkey tetrazzini and smile and say thank you when she puts the tiramisu you don't even care for in front of you—*I don't want to hurt her feelings, and I've already strayed this far.*

Every time you eat when you're not hungry, eat too much, or feel like kicking yourself for having eaten the wrong thing, think about what occurred immediately before the food went into your mouth.

Maybe it was an emotional trigger—a fight with your spouse or a day when everything was running late. It could have been a situation-based trigger—your kid ordered fries but didn't finish them, or you passed by a delicious-looking cupcake display. Whatever they are, triggers kick off a line of thinking that might go like this: *I can't believe I went in and bought a cupcake and ate it on my way out the door. I really screwed up my diet, so I might as well eat whatever I want for the rest of the day and get back on the diet tomorrow.*

If you find yourself struggling with temptation as you progress through the 7 *Years Younger Anti-Aging Breakthrough Diet*, try to pinpoint the triggering thoughts that are sending you down the wrong path. Identify the factors that push you to eat when it's not mealtime or reach for a candy bar instead of a fruit cup, or tempt you to ignore the 7 Years Younger Meal Plan "just this one time." These reasons are your saboteurs.

If you've lost weight in the past and gained it back, and especially if you've gone through the experience several times, you should consider spending a few days or longer on "brain training" before starting the 7 *Years Younger Anti-Aging Breakthrough Diet*. This step has been proven to be a critical part of success. For example, when dieters visit the Beck Institute for weight-loss guidance, they don't start on their diet of choice for up to two weeks. They first start training their brains against sabotage thinking. "Identifying your sabotaging thoughts is crucial," says Bussis, "and responding to them is a skill that you can use for a lifetime to keep excess weight off permanently."

Take a look at your 7 Years Younger Diet Pledge for clues. What are some of the things you wanted to achieve, and what did you identify as obstacles along the way? Take a few minutes to make a list of all the reasons you'd like to lose weight—e.g., you want to get back your youthful energy, you want to have fun buying clothes again, you want to be a good role model for your kids, you don't want the same health problems

Shawna Doyle
"I want to set a good example"

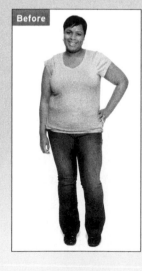

Before

Age
36

Height
5'8"

Weight lost
19 lbs.

Inches lost
9¼ in.

STRUGGLES IN PAST DIETING HISTORY "I'm an emotional eater, and when something went wrong, I'd go to food. 7 Years Younger taught me how to 'recalculate.'"

WHY 7YY "I want to set a good example for my daughters so that they can be healthy and fit. This is the diet that makes it happen, and it really appealed to me because it's all about eating real food."

SUCCESS SECRET "Turning everyday activities into a form of exercise."

PROUDEST OF "Sticking to a workout regimen."

FAVORITE 7YY RECIPE "Turkey-Feta Burgers [page 258]."

BEST ADVICE FOR OTHER DIETERS "Aim to do your personal best, and you will succeed."

Want to be a panelist for a future 7 Years Younger plan? Sign up at 7yearsyounger.com/panelist to be considered.

that Dad has, you want to be able to see your feet when you dance with your daughter at her wedding. Write them all down, no matter how trivial they seem, and put them in visible places that will keep you mentally aware of them—for example, on the wallpaper of your computer screen or posted on the refrigerator door. These written responses are your tools for combating sabotaging thoughts that are likely to arise while you're dieting. Panelist Jeanne Fishwick kept her reminders on her shopping bags so she wouldn't be tempted at the grocery store. These reminders can break the cycle of negative thoughts by bringing to mind all the positive reasons that you have for sticking with a healthy lifestyle. Writing them down is important; making commitments in writing helps keep you psychologically motivated. Bussis counsels dieters to read their reminders aloud at least twice a day until they can't hear their saboteurs anymore. It's not overkill, she says—rather, it is the key to success.

The Pen Is Mightier Than the Mouth

The lower your anxiety level, the greater your capacity for resilience and the less likely it is that you'll self-soothe with food, says Bruce Rabin, M.D., professor of psychiatry at the University of Pittsburgh School of Medicine. But how do you make this equation work in your life? Through writing.

Writing exercises, says Dr. Rabin, help create clarity and reduce anxiety. When you have less anxiety, you have more willpower to resist emotional eating. His technique: Find a quiet place where you won't be disturbed for 15 minutes. Write continuously about something that's bothering you. If you run out of things to write about, just repeat yourself. Don't worry about grammar, and don't stop to read what you've written. At the end of 15 minutes, tear up the piece of paper and toss it out.

"People feel calmer afterward," he says. "Negative thoughts seem to float to the back of the brain."

Practice responses to the triggers that initiate sabotage thinking. For example, when you have an irritating phone conversation with your mother that drives you to the freezer door (as usual), say aloud, "An argument with my mother is no reason to gain weight!" Your written reasons for why you want to slim down are positive reinforcements that you can call on to defeat a trigger.

You can use the same technique to help turn the behavioral changes we described in Chapter 3 into a new healthy habit. For example, if eating on the run is a tough habit for you to break, examine what is causing it to happen. Maybe you don't have enough time to sit down and eat a good breakfast in the morning because you'd rather get an extra 10 minutes of sleep. First, identify in writing the root cause of the problem: *I eat breakfast on the run because I can't get out of bed in the morning.* Then

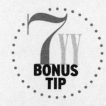

A Strategy for the Long Haul

It seems that keeping up with the losers is a way to stay one yourself. Researchers at Kaiser Permanente tracked 348 successful dieters to find out how they would fare keeping in touch with each other. They found that those who logged on to a diet and fitness website at least once a month for two and a half years after they lost weight kept off more pounds than those who dropped out earlier or signed on less often. Unlike a friend who might stray or get bored, you can always count on a website to be there, explain the researchers, which helps dieters stay committed. Choose an interactive site, such as sparkpeople.com or our own 7 Years Younger online community at 7yearsyounger.com.

resolve to make a change that will work for your lifestyle and also allow you to create a new habit: *I will not push the Snooze button on my alarm clock and will get right out of bed.* In this scenario, when the alarm goes off in the morning and you awaken with a yawn, you'll already have a plan to keep you from hitting that Snooze button.

Letting Go of Emotional Eating

We are all familiar with the triggers of emotional eating: anger, boredom, loneliness, guilt, sadness, rejection, bad hair days. Lots of us, at one time or another, have reacted to our emotions through a jumbo bag of corn chips or a pint of double-fudge ice cream. Research confirms that many people have trouble fighting the scale because when things go awry, their chosen form of therapy is found in the kitchen.

Part of breaking the emotional-eating habit is identifying the triggers that commonly lead you to turn to food. That awareness may help you pause and, in just that short time, make a conscious effort to find something else to comfort yourself.

When you find yourself reaching for something to eat, ask yourself if you are really, truly hungry. How do you know? Physical hunger comes on gradually, but emotional hunger is more immediate—you need a quick fix, and you probably don't care whether that fix fits into your larger health goals. So before you snack, think about whether there is something else you could do to make the craving go away—anything from sipping some water to taking a quick walk that will physically remove you from the trigger zone. If you still want to eat after you've tried distracting yourself, then be prepared with a healthy option to munch on so that you don't hit the diet wreckers.

There are different types of emotional eaters, and different coping strategies work for various types. Read these descriptions and see if any of them apply to you. If so, try the following mind-changing tactics.

The People-Pleaser

Did you buy six boxes of Girl Scout cookies this year because you just couldn't say no to the world's cutest 7-year-old in a Brownie uniform? Did you say yes to a piece of wedding cake because it was handed to you by the bride's mother and you didn't want to be impolite? Do you say OK to ordering in pepperoni pizza for the lunchtime business meeting in the name of being a team player or not wanting to be the odd man out, even though you'd rather have ordered a salad?

If this sounds like you, you feel the need to please others, even if it means eating food that you don't necessarily want in order to follow the crowd. Psychologists even have a name for the condition: sociotropy. Case Western Reserve University researchers demonstrated how this works by screening a group of volunteers for their "gotta be nice" qualities. They invited them to a meeting with a "staff member" (in real life, an actor) who casually passed around a bowl of M&M's after taking a handful himself. When the bowl came their way, students who'd scored high on the sociotropy scale dug in, taking more than the students who were less concerned with others' comfort or with matching how many the actor ate. "They didn't want to make him feel bad by eating fewer," explained researcher Julie Exline, Ph.D.

We often eat more when we're around people who are eating a lot. It's one of the reasons studies show that people whose friends are overweight are more likely to be heavy themselves. "If you have a people-pleasing personality on top of that, you'll feel even more pressured to follow others," says Exline.

The trouble is that overeating is often followed by depression, and not just because you can't zip your jeans. "When your motivation is to please other people, you're letting them tell you what's important to you," says Exline, and that starts eating at you. "I describe it as 'silencing your own voice.'" Here's how to push back:

Ask the EXPERT

Samantha B. Cassetty, M.S., R.D.
Nutrition Director, GHRI

Q *I'm having a really rough week emotionally, and it's starting to get to me—and the diet. What can I do to stay on track?*

Samantha says: Many people fall into this trap, but let me ask you this: When was the last time you felt less angry at yourself or less depressed after having half a box of cookies or a bag of chips? This isn't a rhetorical question, nor is it meant to make you feel defensive (I hate to think of you judging yourself based on your food choices, and I promise I will never judge you based on what's on your plate). I ask the question to encourage you to have a thoughtful dialogue with yourself. The truth is, food can't calm work stress, mend a broken heart, chase away the blues, or take the place of a friend or anything else. And too often, we wind up feeling worse after overeating (thanks to that critical voice in our heads that tells us we're fat, weak, etc.). The point is that food can only feed one thing: physical hunger. If you're eating for other reasons, identify those reasons and find a suitable replacement. My favorite ways to de-stress include deep breathing (I can do it at my desk!) and planning a night out with friends. Squeezing in a workout helps me, too. Praying and listening to music are other popular ways to manage an overloaded to-do list. Pages 135-137 offer more meaningful ways to feed your soul without eating a thing.

Q *My family loves sweets, and I noticed that dark chocolate is on the plan. But I'm worried that if I keep a bag of chocolate in the house, I'll never be able to stop at one piece. What should I do?*

Samantha says: Trust your gut and go cold turkey. Some people do very well with a moderate approach to sweets. For them, knowing there's some chocolate on the plan provides enough pleasure to shore up their willpower and keep them from bingeing on a king-size candy bar. For others, though—and it sounds as if this might be you—this tactic may require too much self-control. In this case, it's easier and less tempting to declare chocolate off-limits.

Consider what *you* want If you're not truly hungry, "lay on the praise, then state your boundary," suggests Karen R. Koenig, a psychotherapist and author of *Nice Girls Finish Fat*. You might say, "Those pastries look delicious, but I'm so stuffed from lunch that I'm going to take a pass." Ask coworkers to order a big salad to share along with the pizza, or request the menu and order yourself a lower-calorie entrée from the same take-out spot. As for the cute Girl Scout, give her a big smile and the money for a box of cookies—or six—and tell her to donate the cookies to a food drive or homeless shelter.

De-nice yourself—a little "Changing isn't as hard as you may think," says Koenig. "It's really about learning a new life skill." Practice by giving a polite but firm no in nonfood situations, such as to the telemarketer who is trying to get you to switch your Internet provider, then work your way up to refusing staffers who are offering you a free taste in the supermarket and coworkers who are pushing another piece of pizza in your direction. You are not going to insult anybody by making decisions that honor your body. Keep reminding yourself of that, and you should be able to turn down cousin Kathy's offer of a second helping of sweet potato pie at Thanksgiving dinner.

The Thrill-Seeker

You're bored with a monotonous task at work, so you head for the vending machine in search of a bag of chips or a candy bar, or maybe both. What you're probably really looking for is a shot of dopamine, says Susan Carnell, Ph.D., research associate at New York Obesity Nutrition Research Center, St. Luke's–Roosevelt Hospital. Dopamine is the brain chemical that drives excitement, pleasure, and motivation—including the excitement and pleasure that motivate you to eat when you're not even hungry. "The dopamine system evolved with the very purpose of making adaptive things like eating feel rewarding so we wouldn't forget to do them," says Carnell.

Ask the EXPERT

Samantha B. Cassetty, M.S., R.D.
Nutrition Director, GHRI

Q *When I've tried dieting before, I've usually lost weight for the first few weeks but then seen my results slow down. What can I do when I hit a diet plateau?*

Samantha says: We've all been there! First, do a reality check. Have you really hit a plateau, or is it possible that you're at a healthy weight? Remember that your stay-young weight isn't about fitting into your high school prom dress—it's about finding the number on the scale that's both healthy and sustainable. If you've seen measurable improvements—pounds shed, inches gone, blood pressure lowered, cholesterol down—this may be a good weight for you.

If you've truly hit a plateau, reinstate your food journal. Maybe too many snacks or sweets have crept back onto your menu, or you're taking too many mindless bites while preparing dinner. Perhaps you've been dipping into the office candy bowl. Using the food diary will help you spot these problems.

If you've taken a few too many passes on your workouts, find a new class or song list to inspire you. Have you fallen into a fitness rut? Try something new to mix things up. Shaking it up from time to time makes your muscles work harder to adapt, and that helps torch more calories.

A final tip: Try using the Jumpstart Week 1 menu as a way to kick-start your weight loss again and firm up your 7 Years Younger routine.

Recent studies have found that ingesting fatty and sugary foods sparks dopamine production in the brain in much the same way heroin or other illegal drugs do, lighting up the neural reward center in imaging studies. "It's just a matter of degree," says Carnell. "Food gives a relatively mild high compared to skydiving and heroin. But it's the easiest route to reward."

There isn't a lot of research on boredom eating, but a small study conducted at Bowling Green State University hints at how prevalent it is. In the study, 139 young men and women reported eating out of boredom more than out of other emotional states linked to overindulging, such as anxiety and depression.

Other studies have approached boredom from a slightly different direction and found a connection between having what scientists call a "novelty-seeking personality" and being overweight. This personality type also has great trouble losing weight. One reason? Overeating is the same as any novelty-seeking addiction. But there are plenty of things that you can do to spice up your life that don't involve hitting the fridge:

Seek out a different thrill There really are things more exciting than food. Make a list of all the nonfood activities that might interest you to fill in the boring blanks. These can be little distractions that you can use to break a food-related thought cycle or longer-term projects that might add some variety to your schedule. "To stimulate your neural circuitry, the activity has to be something that makes you feel excited and motivated," says Carnell. For example, sign up for a language class or learn how to play the ukulele. Dopamine is the chemical that fosters learning and memory, so the novelty of doing something new scatters the chemical throughout your brain. It's important to have some activities you can turn to when a craving strikes, like playing a quick game online or going for a

Dieter's Top Tip

She Plans a Week at a Time

Lynn Bunis, 54, says she found the *7 Years Younger Anti-Aging Breakthrough Diet* easy to follow because she is "intentional" about what she eats: "I like to have a plan to follow, so at the start of each week I decide what I'm going to eat each day, do all the shopping, and make sure I'm always ready for the next day."

To Outsmart a Craving

A craving can sometimes be so strong you can practically taste it, and it feels like it just won't go away until you indulge it.

We usually don't crave things like carrots and broccoli. Foods we crave run more along the lines of chips, ice cream, and cupcakes—choices that lean toward fatty, salty, or sweet. It's mouthfeel that you're looking for, even more than stomach feel. If you're going to cave in, try going for food with a similar taste and texture yet with many fewer calories. Here are some examples:

- **Nachos** A plateful with the works can have 1,520 calories and 100 grams of fat. Kill the craving for just 190 calories and 8 grams of fat by filling a crispy taco shell with refried beans, reduced-fat Cheddar cheese, lettuce, tomato, and salsa. You win by saving 1,330 calories and 92 grams of fat.

- **Pizza** A single slice of four-cheese pizza can cost you 330 calories and 11 grams of fat. But if you take half of a whole wheat pita and top it with chopped tomatoes, some shredded light mozzarella cheese, and some basil and oregano, you can satisfy that pizza craving for 196 calories and 8 grams of fat. You win by saving 134 calories and 3 grams of fat.

- **Loaded potato skins** An order of loaded potato skins has a frightening 2,040 calories and 131 grams of fat. Forget these exist, but get the same satisfaction with a medium baked potato topped with microwave-steamed broccoli and some reduced-fat Cheddar cheese for just 250 calories and 4 grams of fat. You win by saving 1,790 calories and 127 grams of fat.

- **Chocolate-covered ice cream bar** Just one 5-ounce bar comes in at 290 calories and 20 grams of fat. Get the same mouthfeel and a chocolatey taste: Insert an ice-cream stick into a ripe banana, roll it in a crumbled reduced-fat chocolate wafer, and freeze it for only 78 calories and 1 gram of fat. You win by saving 212 calories and 19 grams of fat.

- **Apple pie** A slice of homemade apple pie is around 411 calories and 19 grams of fat. A homemade "baked apple" sprinkled with cinnamon, nutmeg, and brown sugar and microwaved at 70% power until tender (about 3 minutes) is only 108 calories and 0 grams of fat. You win by saving 303 calories and 19 grams of fat.

walk; you could also think about some fun new habits you could add to your life—anything from knitting to joining a local sports league that will give you new ways to fill free time.

Shake up your life regularly Avoid ruts: Do something spontaneous. Grab a coworker and go bowling at lunch; get off the bus at a different stop from your usual one and hoof it the rest of the way to work, checking out the sights you've only seen from a window until now; plan your dream vacation or home-remodeling project in detail, even if it is years in the future. Think about ways to fit something different into your life daily.

You're Overworked, Overwhelmed—And Overeating

These are the three O's that are the downfall of driven women, says psychologist Melissa McCreery, Ph.D., founder of the site toomuchonherplate .com, which explores how women's busy lives contribute to emotional eating and weight gain. The O's can all lead to stress eating. "But there's more to it than stress," says McCreery. "Women who balance many responsibilities

Dieter's Top Tip

Prayer Keeps Her Going

"Hands down, my biggest motivational tool has been prayer," says Shawna Doyle, 36, a working mother of two, who lost 19 pounds in seven weeks. "I keep motivational affirmations handy at all times. Passages like 'My purpose in writing is to encourage you and assure you that what you are experiencing is part of God's grace for you. Stand firm in this grace' help me get recentered, take a few breaths, drink some water, and continue."

struggle with putting themselves first. It takes time. Food is an easy Band-Aid, while real self-care can be more time-intensive." But solutions come in many sizes, and even small changes may be enough to help you avoid the extra pounds that can come with extra work.

Think "doable" You don't want to add more stress to your life. For example, if you typically walk into the house after work and everyone wants a part of you, take five minutes to transition between work and home. Sit in the car and listen to music, meditate, or play a game on your smartphone. Then take a deep breath before you walk through the door so that you can be ready to face whatever and whoever is waiting for you.

Connect with yourself When you're stressed, take five again—five seconds—before digging into the chocolate ice cream. "Ask yourself what's going on and if there's anything else you want to do besides eat," says McCreery. Make a list of small breaks that don't involve chewing: calling a friend, for example, or tossing a toy for your dog.

Say it out loud Greek researchers found that people who were trying to learn a new skill did better when they spoke to themselves using cue words. When you're stressed, voicing your plan to do something other than eat—"I'm going to sit down and read for five minutes"—will change the direction of your thoughts, says McCreery. "It takes you off autopilot and puts you more in control."

If that doesn't work, instead of blaming yourself, be curious. Think about what caused you to grab for the bag of chips and what you could do differently next time to either keep from problem-solving with food or avoid the situation entirely. Overachievers are smart: Harness your wisdom, and you'll find the answers.

Establish a "thin" mindset

A looming deadline, an upcoming dentist appointment, carting kids around from preschool to the pool to a playdate, or even chasing after a new puppy all day can put stresses on you that diminish your motivation and morale—and your weight-loss efforts.

De-stressing from everyday work and life issues can be a powerful psychological way to help keep your motivation on target. A study at Oregon Health and Science University found that overweight women who performed relaxation techniques such as meditation and yoga lost an average of 10 pounds in a year and a half. And here's the clincher: They weren't even consciously dieting. "We suspect that these techniques helped serve as a buffer to stress, so the women were less likely to overeat," says study author Anne Nebrow, M.D.

When we're relaxed, we are literally putting ourselves in the mode of positive thinking. Reveling in feel-good and proud moments can help you stay true to your weight-loss vows, according to the results of three recent studies. In each study, dieters agreed to make lifestyle changes, but only half of them got instructions on how to use affirmations to encourage themselves, such as: "Each morning, think of something that makes you feel good—playing with your dog, finding a bonus in your paycheck, singing your favorite song (even if it's only to yourself)—and continue to recall that pleasure throughout the day." Or: "If you hit a block in your weight-loss efforts—you're getting bored cooking at home, or you don't like walking in the cold—think of a time of pride, such as your wedding day, your graduation, or the birth of your children."

After a year, those who practiced affirmations walked an average of 3.4 more miles a week and burned more calories than a group of dieters who didn't use affirmations. "Recalling accomplishments empowers you to confront challenges," explains researcher Mary E. Charlson, M.D., of Weill Cornell Medical College in New York City.

Visualization works just like affirmations. To improve your eating habits, try this technique used in an experiment at McGill University: Those who made a plan to consume more fruit committed their pledge to paper, pictured themselves carrying the fruit out of the store, and could also see themselves preparing it. The payoff? They were twice as successful at keeping their pledge as people who simply resolved to eat more fruit.

You've already taken the 7 Years Younger Diet Pledge, so you're half-way there.

Activate Your Anti-Aging Diet Now!

1 **Examine your relationship with food** If you've been on more diets than you can count, it's time to give yourself permission to recalibrate your mental attitude about food. Take some time to think about whether you are eating more often because you're physically hungry or for some other reason. Consider whether there are other things you could do besides snack that might address the bigger picture.

2 **Get in touch with your emotional triggers** Awareness of the emotions that drive you to eat when you're not really hungry will help you pause and find something else to comfort you.

3 **Practice stress reduction** Stress can eat away at your morale and destroy your motivation to stay with your diet. Stress-reduction techniques such as yoga, affirmations, and visualization are all strategies proven to work. If stress is your diet enemy, find a technique that suits you and practice it.

For expert anti-aging beauty advice, get our free special report 40 Best Anti-Aging Beauty Secrets at 7yearsyounger.com/antiagingsecrets.

Chapter 5

A Firming Strategy

Ask just about any expert what matters most when it comes to maintaining health and a youthful appearance, and the answer will be the same: exercise. However, the feel-good-about-yourself glow you get from an active lifestyle extends way beyond the boost you feel when someone says you look smashing in your skinny jeans or mistakes you for your grown daughter's sister. Getting regular and consistent exercise is not only age-defying, but also life-extending. A recent study found that a physically active 20-year-old should outlive a same-age couch potato by anywhere from 2½ to 5 years. This is why movement is a key component of the 7 *Years Younger Anti-Aging Breakthrough Diet*. It's not just that weight loss is made easier by exercise or that exercise is essential for keeping weight off. To fight aging, you also want to get and keep your muscles firm. So on the 7 *Years Younger Anti-Aging Breakthrough Diet*, you're going to learn how to have a blast while you move, move, move!

Once you hit age 30, experts say you should get into activities that target all the key areas essential to maintaining vitality and independence as one decade leads to another: balance, endurance, flexibility, and strength. This is what you should strive for on the 7 *Years Younger Anti-Aging Breakthrough Diet*. The kinds of physical activities we're asking you to engage in aren't your typical high-intensity, hour-long workouts! Our plan is all about sustained movement done at frequent intervals. Here's why each of the four pillars of exercise mentioned above is important.

1 **Balance** Physical activity that helps maintain balance, such as ballet, Pilates, yoga, and tai chi, is critical because the small bones in the inner ear, which govern our equilibrium, begin to lose their function as we age. As a result, our balance starts to get out of whack. Avoiding the "clumsiness" that can accompany advancing years is crucial to preventing accidents such as falls, which are the leading cause of bone breaks in elderly Americans.

2 **Endurance** Studies show that aerobic exercise (often referred to as cardio or endurance exercise) has myriad age-defying benefits. Why? Well, the harder you work out, the more energy you use and the more calories you burn. (See the chart on pages 154–155.) Aerobic exercise can also help lower blood pressure. It improves your body's ability to take in and use oxygen and to ferry glucose from the bloodstream into your cells for fuel, a key element in preventing diabetes. And the boost it gives your circulation is awesome for your skin.

3 **Strength training** Lifting weights on a steady basis produces measurable increases in bone density and the strength and size of your muscles. The more muscle you have, the more calories you burn and the less body fat you're likely to store. Strength training is also integral to reducing some of the biggest effects of aging, such as low muscle tone and a slower metabolism.

4 **Flexibility** "Use it or lose it" is the perfect adage to describe what happens when you don't give any thought to stretching your muscles on a regular basis. We lose flexibility as we age. If you don't make a conscious effort to stretch your muscles—say, to reach high cabinets, or extend your hamstrings as if you're touching your toes when picking things up off the ground—your muscles will lose their elasticity. Weak and stiff muscles make you more prone to injury. There's no reason for this to happen, because stretching is something you can do anytime and anywhere.

Why Movement Matters

A sedentary lifestyle accelerates the aging process and can lead to a cascade of age-related health problems. According to Alpa V. Patel, Ph.D., who has studied the health risks associated with too much sitting, it can have a negative impact on your cholesterol, triglycerides, blood pressure, blood sugar, and weight. On the other hand, exercise has the opposite effect. Studies show it discourages the formation of blood clots, shrinks dangerous abdominal fat, and helps reverse age-related losses in muscle mass, bone strength, heart-lung capacity, and flexibility.

Other studies show that people who are more active in midlife stay in

Dieter's Top Tip

Exercise to Energize

"I was an exercise skeptic, thinking that exercise wouldn't lift my mood or give me energy," says Elizabeth Worthy, who worked two 4-plus-mile walks into her day when she decided to stop taking the subway to and from work. "I was so wrong." She lost 11 pounds in just seven weeks, and she's still going.

Malaika Adero
"My dance partners took notice!"

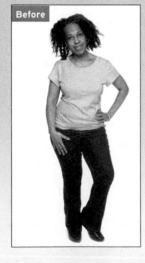

Before

Age
56

Height
5'3"

Weight lost
8 lbs.

Inches lost
¼ in.

STRUGGLES IN PAST DIETING HISTORY "Slipping into bad eating habits when I was busy, such as eating out too much."

WHY 7YY Malaika was drawn to the 7 *Years Younger Anti-Aging Breakthrough Diet* because it appealed to her holistic interest in health. "I liked that it included fitness and healthy food and that it was flexible and sustainable. High blood pressure runs in my family and my community, and I don't want to get it."

SUCCESS SECRET Keeping a food journal. "I found out that eating well means eating quality food in the right quantity," she observes. "It never occurred to me that frozen waffles could be a diet food. When I saw that I could cook dinner a day ahead of time, I ran with it!"

A regular exerciser, Malaika also liked the physical changes that allowed her to enjoy her twice-weekly dance workouts even more. She already had good muscle tone, but she noticed the pain in her knees diminishing as she dropped weight on the program. Plus, "my dance partners definitely took notice that I came down in weight."

PROUDEST OF "The fact that I don't weigh and measure myself. It's enough for me that I feel better and see the changes in my clothes."

FAVORITE 7YY RECIPE "I don't eat red meat, so I enjoyed the Chipotle Lunch (page 228), which is tasty. And since roast chicken with salad is among my favorite dinners, I also liked the mini recipes that were based on buying a rotisserie chicken."

BEST ADVICE FOR OTHER DIETERS "Eat for your overall health and well-being and not to try to live up to the image of others. 'Don't be cheap with your stomach' is a quote from my godparent."

Want to be a panelist for a future 7 Years Younger plan? Sign up at 7yearsyounger.com/panelist to be considered.

better shape as they grow older than people who remain sedentary. No surprise there, of course, but here's the inspiring result: British research found it doesn't take much to gain the benefits. The women in the study were exercising just five or more times a month—proof that even a little exercise is better than no exercise at all.

Here's yet one more reason not to be a slouch: Being active can help make dieting easier by giving you more self-control. In a review, Harvard researchers hypothesized that exercise induces changes in the area of the brain that governs willpower. Think of what your brain tries to make you do when you detect something yummy as you stroll by the bakery—it makes you want to eat what you see in the window, even if you weren't hungry for it a moment ago. But exercise helps strengthen your mental willpower so you can walk by without giving the confections a single thought. As a result, you'll make better food choices.

If you must sit for hours on a daily basis, don't despair. Even if you've never exercised a day in your adult life, you can make up for lost time. A Swedish study that followed more than 2,200 men between the ages of 52 and 80 found that those who increased their activity level from being the equivalent of a casual walker to spending at least three hours a week engaged in endurance activities (such as playing sports or gardening) cut their mortality rate to half that of those who stayed on the sofa.

This doesn't mean you have to run a half-marathon, spin yourself to exhaustion, or step-climb yourself to nowhere fast in order to like what you see in the mirror when you wake up in the morning. In order to enjoy the lasting results of exercise, you need to find a natural way to integrate it so that you actually enjoy it. Ultimately, the goal of the *7 Years Younger Anti-Aging Breakthrough Diet* is to get you engaging in 30 minutes of exercise five times a week—the amount experts say it takes to be fit. You won't even have to do all 30 minutes at once; studies show that three 10-minute bouts are just as effective.

Ask the EXPERT

Jennifer Cook
Senior Executive Editor, *Good Housekeeping*

Q *Is it really necessary to warm up before and cool down after exercise?*

Jenny says: This is a tough one, since the research is mixed on the health benefits of warm-ups and cooldowns. But when I've asked fitness experts if they think these things are beneficial, they've usually said yes. There's more scientific support for warming up—it slowly raises your body temperature, warms your muscles so you don't hurt yourself, and prepares your joints to go through their full range of motion. Try a dynamic warm-up: gentle aerobic exercise like walking or cycling slowly, arm circles, and leg swings. As for the cooldown, it may or may not be necessary, but it feels good. Slowing down the pace lets you lower your heart rate gently and may help prevent dizziness, and stretching while your muscles are warm will boost your flexibility and minimize soreness. And that will make your next workout even better.

Q *I can only exercise on the weekend. What is the best routine for me?*

Jenny says: Since you just have two days, you'll need to take care not to push too hard and get hurt. To avoid this problem and get the most out of your Saturday and Sunday sessions, Richard Cotton, national director of certification at the American College of Sports Medicine, advises boosting your everyday activity from Monday through Friday. Take the stairs, go for brisk lunchtime walks, and park at the back of the lot (see other examples on page 158). On the weekends, do a half hour of cardio and the strength-training routine on pages 166-169 on both days. On Saturdays, ease up a bit and make sure you have a couple of repetitions left in you before finishing each move. On Sundays, you can push yourself harder, since you'll have a full five days to recover. Or, plan an active family outing (like a long hike) instead.

Joining a gym if you don't think you'll actually go or lacing up a pair of running shoes to hit the pavement when you haven't done so in years could set you up for failure. Research shows that taking small steps, not giant leaps, leads to greater strides toward reaching your weight-loss goal and making fitness a habit. Panelist Winston Leung tried to offset his sedentary day life by going to the gym after work. "But that didn't work, because working out made me hungry and I'd actually eat more," he reports. What ultimately helped him was changing his focus to walking more throughout the day and hopping on his elliptical trainer at home at night. That's what weight-loss and exercise expert Lesley D. Lutes, Ph.D., discovered when she and a team of colleagues from East Carolina University asked a group of dieters to commit to an exercise almost everyone can do—walking. Women in the study gradually increased their daily steps while they simultaneously reduced calories and added healthier food to their diets at an equally gradual rate. The women kept at it for three months—slowly increasing their activity level, eating healthier, and even phoning each other for motivation and inspiration. The result? Lutes found that success came from adding just an extra 500 to 1,000 steps a day or every few days; what's more, these simple steps played a pivotal role in turning walking into a habitual form of exercise. "Truth is, only 10% of people go to the gym regularly," she says. "The other 90% have to make physical activity happen through other methods." If you do it properly, you can get the same quality of exercise as a workout maven without ever crossing the threshold of a gym.

The women in the study achieved what Lutes called "clinically significant weight loss"—an average of nearly 9 pounds. Even better, they continued to lose, an average of another 8 pounds when the researchers checked in again three and six months later.

"We are finding that initially, making changes in diet alone will lead to weight loss," says Lutes, "but physical activity is the key component to long-term weight-loss maintenance. Without it, you're going to see the weight go back up."

The Road to Fitness

This is your road map to integrating the four important pillars of fitness into your life. Your ultimate goal should be to engage in 30 minutes of heart-pumping exercise five times a week. You can do the 30 minutes all at once, or you can break it into three 10-minute sessions. If you are new to exercise or you haven't been seriously focused on it for a long time, this approach will help you get in shape as you shed pounds.

Warm up, cool down Don't start any exercise cold. If you're walking, start out slowly for two to four minutes before picking up the pace. If you're jogging, start out walking for the same amount of time. When you've finished, slow down your walking to help slow down your heart. Walk around to loosen up your muscles before doing toning or stretching exercises.

Start moving Once you're warmed up, pick up the pace until your heart is pumping. You should be moving briskly enough that your breathing picks up, but not so fast that you can't catch your breath. If you're a beginner, you can start out by just walking as far as is comfortable for you and gradually add more distance—500-step increments is a good goal—until you reach 30 minutes. Then feel free to keep going—the farther, the better. If you already participate in other aerobic activities, like spinning or Zumba class, you can still try to fit walking into your day. Remember: The more active you are, the more calories you'll burn.

Step it up A part of your goal is to move more throughout the day. Set a goal for yourself to take 10,000 steps a day, and build up to that no matter what your current step count is. Use a pedometer; research shows pedometer users make the biggest strides. (You'll find tips on how to use a pedometer on page 156.)

Tone Take your measurements at the same time as you do your official weigh-in at the start of your diet. Measure your waist, stomach, hips, chest, and thighs. Start doing toning and strengthening exercises, such as those we recommend on pages 166–169. Take your measurements and log them in your diet journal every week; you'll feel great as you start being able to measure the difference.

Get flexible Unless you've mastered yoga, we can all improve in this area! Take the flexibility test on page 176. Do stretching exercises or sign up for a beginners' yoga class or any class that focuses on stretching and flexibility. This will also help you maintain or improve your balance as you get older.

As you're figuring out the best ways to integrate movement into your day, remember to listen to your body. Don't try to do too much too fast.

If your body starts talking back—say, with prolonged muscle soreness, intense fatigue, or uncomfortable pressure—back off a little until you're more comfortable. But don't be afraid to challenge yourself. You'll be amazed at how good you feel when you start moving, and you're going to love the reward!

The Burn Cycle: How Activity Adds Up

The number of calories you will actually burn depends on you—your age, your gender, the amount of fat you're carrying around, how efficiently you move, and even your environment. Of course, it is difficult to quantify such vast differences from person to person, but science has come up with a way. It's called the metabolic equivalent, or what scientists call MET.

MET is a standardized value scientists around the world have been using for the last 20 years to measure the energy output for hundreds of specific activities. In scientific terms, no matter how athletic you are or what you weigh, the amount of energy you expend at rest is roughly 1 MET, or 1 calorie per every kilo of your body weight. Translated, that is 1 calorie for every 2.2 pounds of weight. Stand up, and you're now burning 1.3 MET. Start fidgeting, and you're burning 1.8 MET. Open the door and start walking, and your MET rises to 3.5. It's pretty much the same for everybody. The difference, however, is based on your weight.

As an example, let's look at a 10-minute mile. If a 125-pound woman and a 180-pound man go running together at a pace of 6 miles per hour, all things being equal, she will burn roughly 556 calories an hour, while he'll burn roughly 801—a prime example of why men can often get away with eating more than women.

The formula for figuring it out is simple arithmetic that takes just seconds to do if you use the calculator on your smartphone or computer:

Your weight divided by 2.2 multiplied by MET.

Activity	MET	Duration	Cal. Burned
Backpacking	7.0	4 hrs.	1,781
Bowling	3.8	2 hrs.	484
Breast-feeding	2.0	2 hrs.	255
Making the bed	2.5	10 mins.	27
Child care, intermittent active time	2.0	8 hrs.	1,018
Cleaning the house	3.3	1.5 hrs.	315
Cycling (10 mph)	4.0	30 mins.	127
Dancing: disco, line, country	7.8	1 hr.	496
Using elliptical trainer, moderate speed	5.0	30 mins.	159
Food shopping	2.3	1 hr.	146
Gardening, moderate intensity	5.0	1 hr.	318
Giving the dog a bath	3.5	30 mins.	111
Golf, carrying bags	4.8	4 hrs.	1,221
Hatha yoga	2.5	1 hr.	159
Horseback riding	5.5	1 hr.	350
Jogging, 15 mins (4-mph pace)	6.0	30 mins.	190
Jumping rope	11.0	10 mins.	116
Kayaking	5.0	1 hr.	318
Moving furniture around or carrying heavy bags	5.8	15 mins.	92
Mowing the lawn with a power mower	5.5	1 hr.	350
Office work	1.5	8 hrs.	763
Painting a room	3.3	3 hrs.	630

Or, a 140-pound person (140 divided by 2.2 = 63.6) running a 10-minute-mile pace at 9.8 MET (times 9.8) will burn roughly 624 calories an hour, or roughly 104 calories per mile, give or take a few. That's how you end up with the generalization that running a mile burns around 100 calories.

A difference of 10 or 20 calories here and there doesn't seem like a lot, but it adds up over the course of weeks, months, and years. The above chart gives calorie expenditure for the amount of time you're likely to

Activity	MET	Duration	Cal. Burned
Pilates	3.0	1 hr.	191
Playing active games with the kids	5.8	1 hr.	369
Playing pool	2.5	1 hr.	159
Power yoga	4.0	1 hr.	255
Resistance training	6.0	1 hr.	381
Running, 6-mph pace	9.8	30 mins.	312
Scuba diving	7.0	1 hr.	445
Sitting quietly	1.0	1 hr.	64
Skiing, cross-country	9.0	1 hr.	572
Skiing, downhill	5.3	1 hr.	337
Sleeping	.95	8 hrs.	484
Standing, doing nothing	1.3	1 hr.	82
Standing, doing something	1.8	1 hr.	114
Stationary bike, moderate effort (30 to 50 watts)	3.5	30 mins.	111
Swimming, slow to moderate speed	5.8	20 mins.	123
Tennis, singles	7.3	1 hr.	464
Typing on the computer	1.3	1 hr.	82
Walking, brisk pace (3.5 mph)	4.3	30 mins.	137
Walking, moderate pace (3 mph)	3.5	30 mins.	111
Washing the car	3.5	30 mins.	111
Watching TV	1.0	2 hrs.	128
Yard work, moderate intensity	4.0	2 hrs.	509

Source: Compendium of Physical Activities 2011

engage in certain activities throughout the day or week (based on a 140-pound man or woman) and the activity's metabolic equivalent.

Getting Fit One Step at a Time

Walking is one of the easiest forms of exercise. You can do it anywhere, for as much time as you have available, and you don't need anything beyond a good pair of sneakers or running shoes to do it. No wonder

Pedometer: A Must-Have Accessory

A pedometer can be as important to your everyday life as your watch and the keys to the car. This inexpensive little device, which snaps onto your belt or waistband, measures and records the number of steps you take (often also calculating the number of calories being expended) throughout the day. A review of more than two dozen studies involving 2,767 people associated pedometer use with "significant increases in physical activity and significant decreases in body mass index and blood pressure."

Studies show that left to their own estimates of what's fast enough, many people aren't getting the fitness boost out of their movement they think they are. To find the best speed, researchers from San Diego State University measured energy output as 97 people walked on a treadmill, then translated their speed to a formula everyone can use. The minimum pace? About 100 steps a minute. You can check your pace with your pedometer.

Research shows that pedometer users take about 2,500 more steps a day—a little over a mile—than people who don't carry one. In weight-loss terms, that is equal to 10 pounds a year! "It is the best motivational tool around," says exercise expert Lutes of East Carolina University. "It's visual feedback. It also helps make walking habit-forming."

Pedometers are easy to use, and you don't have to buy anything fancy. For $30 or even less, you can get a dependable, comfortable, and simple-to-operate pedometer with a built-in clock so you don't lose track of time. All you do is measure your stride, enter it into the gadget's memory, push a button, and off you go.

Our panelists used the Omron Pedometer; it's straightforward to set up and can be synced through the integrated USB connection to the website omronfitness.com. There, users can track daily progress and set calorie, step, and distance goals. The same metrics are viewable on the pedometer itself, which can be carried in a pocket or clipped to a belt.

walking has the distinction of having the lowest dropout rate of any form of exercise. To get the most benefit, you should aim to spend the majority of your time moving at a good clip. For some people, that's just short of breaking into a jog. For others, it can be a few notches above a stroll. Move at the fastest pace you can handle. It's good to start out slowly, for two to three minutes at most, as this will help loosen and warm you up, but then you have to move it—with arms pumping and at a pace that makes you breathe hard. If you're walking and you can easily carry on a conversation, then you aren't moving fast enough!

Walking is essential, not just as a weight-loss aid and to exercise your heart, but also as an anti-aging strategy. Once bone mass peaks, you can start to lose it at a rate of about 1% to 2% per year. But regular weight-bearing activity that puts pressure on your legs, such as walking or jogging, actually increases bone density in your lower body.

Harvard researchers discovered another benefit: Walking can have a positive effect on genes that influence weight gain or loss. Researchers measured these "fat genes" in 12,000 men and women and then looked at their fat-to-muscle ratios and exercise patterns. The motivating math: Walking briskly for an hour a day can halve the damage weight-promoting genes do to your fat-to-muscle ratio by curbing their activity. However, the reverse is also true, says study author Qibin Qi, Ph.D. Hours spent watching TV can up the activity of the same genes, with a 25% increase in their fat-storing ability for every two hours of daily tube time.

In order to get the most out of your walking, try this body-toning walking style to get your heart pumping:

- Keep your face forward—no looking down. Hold your arms at a 90-degree angle and pump them back and forth, with your hands in loose fists. Stand upright, with your shoulders back and relaxed.

Take a Lap

Here are just a few suggestions of other ways to fit more steps into your life. Try these, but feel free to get creative and make up your own ideas:

- Take one full sweep of the perimeter of the supermarket with your cart, then start shopping
- Pace the room while talking on the phone
- Take a walk around the block after each time you eat, even if you've just had a snack
- Park your car as far away as possible from, instead of close to, the entrance when going to places such as the supermarket or the mall
- Walk instead of drive for all trips that are a mile or less
- Always take the stairs instead of the elevator or escalator, or walk the escalator
- Make one circuit of the mall before you start to browse and shop
- If you work at a desk all day, take a three-minute break every half hour to get up and walk around
- Don't jaywalk; always walk to the farthest corner before crossing the street
- If you commute using public transportation, get off the subway or bus a stop or two before your destination. If you take the train, board the car that will make you walk the farthest
- When you have to stand around and wait (for something or someone), pace back and forth
- Avoid the drive-through at the bank and library; instead, park your car at a distance so you can get in some steps walking back and forth
- Use the restroom one flight up from where you are
- Get more active as a family or with friends. Go to a museum, start a bowling league, or rent a canoe or kayak. Think of fun activities that will get you moving

- Always place your heel down first and let the middle of your foot and your toes follow.

March uphill Choose a hill at least a block long. If you live in the flatlands, step on a treadmill and increase the incline to 4%. No hills, no treadmill? Walk up steps for one minute.

Start out small "You need to set a goal realistic for your lifestyle," says Lutes. "If you now only take 2,000 steps throughout the day, you can't say you're going to start walking for a half hour a day starting on day one, because it's not going to happen. Or at least it is not going to last. Even adding 500 steps to your day is a 25% increase, and that is a lot." Add more steps every day or every few days—whatever is comfortable for you. Try small things, like parking farther away from the entrance when you go shopping or taking the stairs instead of the elevator. You've heard it before, but after a few months, these behaviors will just become a habit that makes the next level of exercise come a little easier.

Then start ramping it up Let's say you now manage about 3,000 steps a day. If you add 500 steps a week, you'll be at five miles a day after three months. If you work up to walking for 30 minutes a day, even if it isn't all at one time, and actively move about throughout the day, you eventually will hit 10,000 steps as if they were nothing.

Take a walk while the coffee brews The best way to maximize your steps is with a daily walk, and the surest way to fit it in may be to do it first thing in the A.M. Just set your alarm to go off a half hour earlier than usual, throw on your walking gear, turn on the coffeemaker, and head out the door. You can get the rest of the family up after you get back—if the smell of the brew hasn't done so already. And here's a bonus: Research shows that when you exercise aerobically on an empty stomach, you can burn 20% more fat without increasing your appetite or eating more throughout the day.

Go the extra steps The whole idea is to step it up whenever and wherever you can. So, instead of sending an e-mail to your colleague five cubicles away, get up and deliver the message in person. Is it really necessary to take the car to the mailbox a block and a half away? Do the kids have to be driven to the school bus when all of you could benefit from the walk?

Make It Aerobic

Aerobic, or endurance, exercise can delay biological aging 10 years or more, increasing the likelihood that you'll stay fit, mobile, and independent as the decades pass. And while the risk of many diseases, from diabetes to cancer to heart disease, increases with age, there is a bounty of evidence suggesting that heart-pumping exercise can help keep them at bay.

These activities are a sampling of exercises that are considered to be moderately aerobic:

- Walking at a pace of 3 mph
- Heavy-duty cleaning
- Fast dancing
- Swimming laps
- Racquetball
- Low-impact aerobics

These activities will give you a more vigorous workout:

- Cross-country skiing
- Running at a pace of 5 mph
- Singles tennis
- High-impact aerobics
- Vigorous calisthenics, such as push-ups or jumping jacks

Even if you've never broken a sweat on the track or taken a spinning class, it's never too late to start reaping the benefits of aerobic exercise.

20-Minute Interval Workout

To get your routine started, try doing this 20-minute interval workout up to five times per week. Use your pedometer to keep track of your steps, and keep plenty of water handy:

- **2 mins.** Warm up
- **1 min.** Walk at moderate speed
- **30 secs.** Walk fast
- **1 min.** Walk at moderate speed
- **1 min.** Walk fast
- **30 secs.** Walk at moderate speed
- **30 secs.** Walk fast
- **1.5 mins.** Walk at moderate speed
- **30 secs.** Walk fast
- **3 mins.** Walk at moderate speed
- **1.5 mins.** Walk fast
- **2 mins.** Walk at moderate speed
- **1 min.** Walk fast
- **2 mins.** Walk at moderate speed
- **2 mins.** Cool down

Researchers from the University of California at Berkeley proved this after finding a group of sedentary postmenopausal women who were willing to hop on a stationary bike and a treadmill as their introduction to aerobic conditioning. They pedaled and walked at aerobic capacity for an hour a day, five days a week. After 12 weeks, they were functioning "as though they were 20 years younger," says researcher George A. Brooks, Ph.D. They experienced improvements in their blood pressure and blood sugar levels and in their ability to take in and use oxygen. Their heart rates dropped to much healthier levels, and their ability to burn fat increased 10%. Now, *that's* incentive! Here are some tips to help you get started on making your exercise aerobic so you can reap similar rewards.

Do intervals Alternating short bursts of all-out effort with longer bouts at a slower steady speed can ramp up your fat-burning capacity tremendously. In one study, researchers divided 45 lean and overweight women into two groups. One group cycled steadily at a moderate speed for 40 minutes, and the other switched between sprinting for eight seconds and light pedaling for 12 seconds—doing what's called "interval training"—over a 20-minute workout. The women doing the intervals lost three times as much fat as the women who exercised at a moderate pace for twice as long. Without changing their diets, the sprinters also dropped an average of 5½ pounds, while the non-sprinters gained a pound.

How does interval training yield these great results? "More muscle fibers get worked during those high-intensity intervals," says Martin Gibala, Ph.D., an exercise physiologist at McMaster University. "When you push hard in a short burst, it reactivates nerve fibers, builds new capillaries, and forces your body to repair the muscle. All of that burns a tremendous number of calories."

There are plenty of enjoyable ways to put more endurance training in your life that do not require you to lace up your sneakers or pull out your workout clothes. Here are some ideas:

Climb the stairway to success It goes without saying that you should always take the stairs instead of the elevator when going up or coming down a few floors. Here's the incentive for doing so: Just three minutes of

The 10-Minute 101-Calorie Burn

Oops, you can't believe you ate the whole thing! When the inevitable happens, don't toss out the diet or get discouraged; just tie on your sneakers and hop to it. Here's how to burn off 101 unwanted calories in just 10 minutes:

- **1 minute:** Lift something heavy just like you would a barbell, curling your arms in toward your chest—7 calories gone
- **3 minutes:** Jump rope—36 calories gone
- **3 minutes:** Do jumping jacks—29 calories gone
- **3 minutes:** Jog in place—another 29 calories gone

That's all there is to it! Whether you want to keep a trigger moment from sending you into a spiral of bad thoughts or you just need a way to get your blood pumping, 10 minutes of sustained exercise is a terrific way to burn calories and keep yourself feeling like you're in control.

stair-climbing every day burns enough calories to prevent the average gain of a half-pound to one and a half pounds for Americans every year. It can also help you live longer. A study at Harvard University found that men who climbed more than 70 flights of stairs a week had an 18% lower early-death rate than men who climbed fewer than 20 flights. That works out to 10 flights a day, not a big deal if you live in a two-story house or work in a multi-floor office building.

Get vertical Keep this in the forefront of your brain: Standers are thinner than sitters. Not only does sitting all day burn fewer calories, but it also slows your metabolism, which gets pokey with age as it is. "As soon as you stand up, you start to activate your body's metabolic engines," says James Levine, M.D., an obesity expert at the Mayo Clinic in Rochester, MN. Never sit when you can stand.

Take commercial breaks You don't have to give up *Modern Family* to fit in some exercise. There are a lot of commercials during a typical TV show—enough, in fact, for you to sneak in a pretty good workout. The workout even has a name: TV Commercial Stepping. Research by Jeremy A. Steeves, Ph.D., of the National Institutes of Health, found that marching in place or walking around the room at a brisk pace during the commercials of 90 minutes of TV offers the same benefits as walking on a treadmill nonstop for 30 minutes. It moved one group of individuals from sedentary to somewhat active status without any other added exercise. To make it work for you, make sure you march briskly, with arms pumping and legs lifted high. Since you're probably wondering: a half-hour program has between eight and 12 minutes of commercial breaks.

As you start working more and more strenuous activity into your day, think of a tough workout as the gift that keeps on giving. When researchers from Appalachian State University in Boone, NC, asked cyclists to bike at a vigorous pace for 45 minutes, they found that the cyclists continued to burn calories post-exercise for the next 14 hours. To maximize your calorie burn—and blast fat—you would need to work up a sweat doing intense cardio, such as a spinning class, for 45 minutes three times a week. Not something you have to jump on right away, but give it a try when you're feeling ambitious!

Get Strong, 20 Minutes at a Time

The sooner you're ready to fit some strength training into your day, the better, because it can help you lose weight faster. When you strengthen your muscles, you're building a calorie-burning machine. In fact, some studies estimate that you burn an additional 35 to 50 calories a day with each pound of muscle you add to your body.

Strength training is a proven way to keep your metabolic rate from dropping with age. Because muscle burns more calories than other types of body tissue, building muscle mass increases your metabolic rate, helping to counteract the 5% loss per decade that accompanies aging. In fact, most of what we recognize as aging is actually muscle loss.

Strength training works by stressing muscle fibers in ways that prompt them to repair and rebuild themselves. Regular sessions of lifting weights or other forms of resistance training promote a continual remodeling of muscle tissue, increasing your calorie-burning ability and toning and tightening your body. As you sculpt your muscles, you'll be building a firm foundation for skin, preventing the appearance of wrinkles, droops, and sags.

Strength training can even slow the aging of your cells. It turns out that structures inside cells called mitochondria, which turn nutrients into energy, tend to operate less effectively as the body ages. Scientists believe this slowdown may be involved in muscle loss. Research also shows that strength-building may boost longevity in other ways. It can help lower blood pressure, build bone, improve mental acuity, and reduce the risk of heart disease, arthritis, and type 2 diabetes.

Ask the EXPERT

Samantha B. Cassetty, M.S., R.D.
Nutrition Director, GHRI

Q *I just logged extra miles on my walk. Is it OK to treat myself to something sweet?*

Samantha says: I wish I could say yes, but the unfortunate truth is that you probably didn't burn as many calories as you suspect, so it's not a good idea to use your workout as a reason to splurge. Let me put it this way: A brisk 30-minute walk burns about half the calories you get in a small portion of cookie dough ice cream. I rest my case.

Q *Help! I've been walking two miles a day for weeks and my weight isn't changing. Why not?*

Samantha says: It may feel like a lot, but that amount of walking, while key to your health, isn't enough to move the needle on the scale. The calorie burn barely covers your daily snack allowance! So if you find yourself saying things like, "I walked two miles today; I earned this piece of chocolate," you're not only negating your walk with that treat, you're eating more calories than you walked off. Take a look at your diet—are there places you might be slipping (like taking too many tastes while cooking or indulging in your kids' fries)? Once you get comfortable on the plan, it's easy to start eyeballing—and over-serving—things like chips, nuts, and cereal. Or, you may have become less vigilant about brown-bagging your lunch or cooking rather than grabbing takeout, which are both key to your success. Another possibility: Your body may simply have adapted to this daily routine and now be burning fewer calories than it used to while doing the same thing. That's why you need to continuously boost your workouts—either by going longer or by working harder. To increase workout intensity, try interval walking (see the plan on page 161) or jogging. You could also try adding hills or stairs. (Just don't change everything at once!) These tweaks to your diet and exercise routine should get the needle on the scale moving again.

7 Years Younger Strengtheners

For this introductory workout, all you need are some comfortable clothes, a bath towel, and a rubber ball about the size of a soccer ball. As promised, there is no gym required. The entire routine takes about 20 minutes and is designed to firm your tummy, thighs, chest, and arms. If strength training is new to you, or if you haven't done it in a while, ease into it—but don't hesitate to keep turning it up a notch as you begin to experience success.

Do 12 reps (one on the left side plus one on the right side equals one rep, where applicable) of each exercise.

Warm-Up (4 minutes)

You need to get your heart rate up, and the quickest way to do it is on a step. Using a step stool or stairs, step up with your right foot, then up with the left, then down with the right and down with the left. After one minute, switch sides to start with the left foot. Repeat both sides again. If you don't have stairs, jog in place or walk briskly around the house.

1. Ab Twist (2 minutes) **Muscles worked** Abs, glutes, and hamstrings

a   b

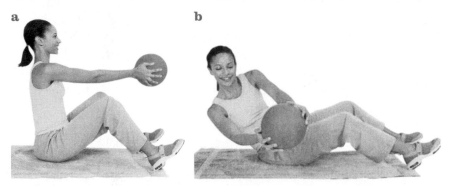

a. **Sit on a towel** on the floor with your feet shoulder-width apart, knees up, and toes pointing up so your feet are resting on your heels. Hold the ball with both hands and extend your arms in front of you.

b. **Slowly lie back,** keeping your abs tucked and tightened. Stop halfway to the floor and twist to the left, reaching toward the floor with the ball. Hold for a beat, then slowly twist to the right, reaching toward the floor. Breathe normally and concentrate on contracting your abs.

2. Wall Squat (2 minutes)
Muscles worked Glutes, hamstrings, and quadriceps

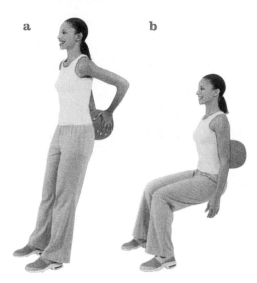

a

b

a. **Stand with your back to the wall** and put the ball in the small of your back. Place your feet shoulder-width apart with toes forward and abs tucked.

b. **Over a count of five,** slowly bend your knees to lower your body until the backs of your thighs (the hamstrings) are almost parallel to the floor. Hold, then squeeze your butt (the glutes) and press back up over a count of five. Keep the ball between your back and the wall throughout the exercise.

3. Back Pull (2 minutes)
Muscles worked Back

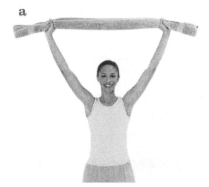

a

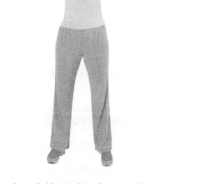

b

a. **Roll the towel lengthwise.** Grasping an end in either hand, raise it over your head with both arms extended.

b. **Inhale, then slowly exhale,** bending your arms and lowering the towel behind your head. Keep tension on the towel as you raise and lower it, but don't tighten your neck.

4. Push-Up (2 minutes)
Muscles worked Chest and arm muscles

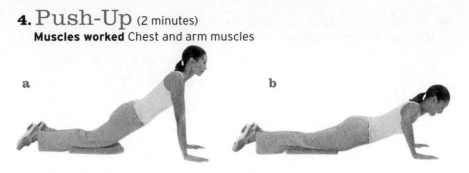

a.   b.

a. **Fold the towel** into a small square and place it under your knees for support. Kneeling on the towel, walk your hands forward, with your fingers spread, until your torso is at a 45-degree incline to the floor. Your hands should be slightly wider than shoulder-width apart.

b. **Tuck your abs as you lower yourself** until you are about two inches from the floor. Squeeze your chest muscles as you press up to the starting position.

5. Bridge (2 minutes)
Muscles worked Abs, glutes, and hamstrings

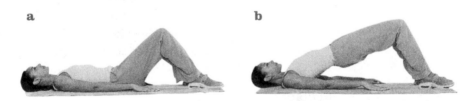

a.   b.

a. **Lie on your back** on a towel with your knees bent, your feet flat on the floor, and your arms at your sides. If you feel tension in your neck, tuck another towel under your head for support.

b. **Inhale, then raise your butt and your lower back** off the floor as you exhale. Keep your back straight and your head and shoulders on the floor. Hold for one count. Slowly release and lower, but don't let your bottom touch the floor until you complete all the reps. Focus on squeezing your glutes at the top of each rep.

6. Hamstring Curl (2 minutes)
Muscles worked Hamstrings, glutes, and lower back

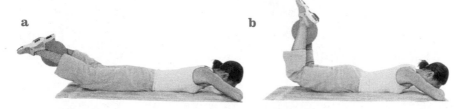

a.

b.

a. **Lie flat on your stomach** on your towel. Place the ball between your lower legs, close to your ankles. Cross your arms and rest your forehead on them. Squeeze the ball and, keeping your legs as straight as possible, lift your knees off the floor as high as possible.

b. **Slowly bend your knees** until your toes are pointing toward the ceiling. Exhale as you curl up and inhale as you release. You should keep your knees off the floor for the entire exercise. If you feel strain in your lower back, rest for a moment and then resume the exercise.

7. Arm Extension (4 minutes)
Muscles worked Triceps

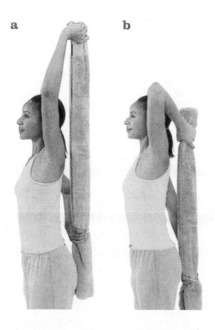

a.

b.

a. **Roll up the towel lengthwise.** Place one end in your left hand. Straighten your left arm directly over your head so the towel dangles behind you. Reach your right arm behind your back and grasp the towel three-quarters of the way down.

b. **Gently pull the towel down with your right arm,** bending your left arm behind your head so your elbow points straight up. Inhale, holding the towel steady. Exhale and extend your left arm back to the starting position, keeping tension on the towel with your right arm. Do 6 reps. Switch arms and repeat.

Improve Your Balance

The payoff of being diligent about your balance is not just in the prevention of falls. Balance can improve your coordination, prevent injuries as you're practicing other forms of exercise, and even boost your posture. Balance training will make you more aware of your body and the way you move, which will help you in all the other areas of fitness you're working on. You can develop your sense of balance—or improve it—and you don't need a special workout to do it. Here are easy ways to sneak balance exercises into your day.

- Stand on one foot, then the other as you brush your teeth.
- While waiting in line, walk in place by putting your feet down from heel to toe.
- Balance on one foot as you put on socks or shoes.
- Hike off-road: Stepping around rocks, over tree roots, and through loose gravel improves your balance.
- Walk forward and backward about 10 steps along a straight line (the edge of a sidewalk or an imaginary line).
- Dance: The forward, backward, and side-to-side movement of most forms of dance develops your equilibrium.

The Number One Flat-Belly Move

The fastest way to a flat tummy is a simple move you probably already know how to do: the bicycle. It's the most effective ab exercise because it activates muscles on the front and sides of your belly and makes them work two to three times harder than a standard crunch. Here's a how-to reminder:

Lie on your back with your knees bent, your feet lifted, and your hands clasped under your head. Extend your right leg straight out while lifting your shoulder blades off the floor, bringing your left knee into your chest and twisting your right armpit toward your left knee. Pause, then switch sides. Do two sets of 15 reps three times a week.

These little exercises might not sound like much, but they can make a real difference in the way you relate to your body.

Multitask Yourself Into a Better Body

We are all so used to trying to do too many things at once—answering e-mails while talking on the phone, watching TV while surfing the Internet, trying to spend quality time with someone while checking our smartphones. But when it comes to your fitness, there is a lot of great multitasking that you can do to squeeze mini tightening exercises into your day, even when you're on the job. Here are some of our favorite options:

Firm and fold Here's an exercise you can do while folding laundry, courtesy of Amanda Russell, a New York City fitness trainer. Put your basket of laundry on the floor rather than on the bed or on a table. Stand with your feet a little wider than shoulder-width apart, toes turned slightly out. Each time you retrieve an item from the basket, slowly bend your knees and lower yourself into a squat. Go as far down as you can while still keeping your back straight. Do not let your knees extend forward past your toes. Slowly rise to a standing position. Repeat until all the laundry is folded.

Do the grocery-bag burn Lugging groceries to and from your car is practically a form of weight-lifting already, so you might as well take advantage of it and give your biceps a workout, which will also help you prevent or get rid of the unflattering scourge of aging—the flabby area underneath your arms. Here's how:

Hold your grocery or shopping bags by the handles the way you would put your hands around a set of dumbbells: palms facing up and elbows by your sides. Bend your arms, slowly lift the bags toward your shoulders, then slowly lower them. Do as many reps as you can, rest, and then do a few more.

Upgrade your twists and turns You can turn practically any natural movement into a mini workout. Here are five we like that you can do every day:

- When you're out walking throughout the course of the day, increase your pace, tighten your glutes and abs, and pump your arms, suggests Ramona Braganza, who trains stars such as Jessica Alba. You'll burn 40 extra calories in 30 minutes!

- Here's an exercise to do while you're waiting at a red light (don't exercise while your car is moving!). Squeeze your lower abdominal muscles and draw your belly button in and up, as if you're trying to squeeze into a pair of tight jeans. Hold until the light turns green or for as long as you can. "This engages the transverse abdominals, which helps sculpt and flatten your stomach," says Los Angeles–based Pilates instructor Jillian Hessel.

- As you climb stairs, grab on to the railing and take them two at a time, pushing down through your heels. This works your bottom extra hard. If you do a lot of stair-climbing during the day, it can add up to some serious calorie burn.

Do some desk-ercise You don't even have to get out of your chair to do these firming exercises. Just slide your chair out from under the desk and kick off your heels (if you're wearing them). This thigh-firmer comes courtesy of trainer Tracey Mallett, creator of the *Get Your Body Back* and *Booty Barre Workout* DVDs:

Sit up straight in your chair with your feet flat on the floor. Grasp the sides of your seat with your hands for support. Slowly lift one foot, with the knee still bent, off the floor about six inches and lower it back down. Do this 10 times, switch legs, and repeat. Next, lift your foot off the floor the same way and quickly pulse your leg up and down for a count of 10. Switch legs and repeat.

Dance the Weight Away

So you say you can dance? Great! Shaking a leg is one of the more fun ways to firm up and slim down. Besides, you'll look and feel sexy doing it. Getting out on the dance floor for just 15 minutes of continuous vigorous moves could burn as many as 110 calories. So don't just watch and tap your foot when the music comes on. Get up and swing (or cha-cha, or waltz).

"What sets dancing apart is how the body responds to music," says Elizabeth Larkam, spokesperson for the American Council on Exercise. The beat makes you want to keep going even though being out of breath to the same extent would make you cut most other aerobic workouts short.

Dancing also offers another anti-aging benefit besides slimming you in all the right places: One study found that people who dance four or more times a week have a 76% lower risk of dementia than those who sit it out. The physical act of doing the fox-trot or the merengue increases blood flow to the brain. Additionally, it requires some mental effort to listen to the music, pick up the beat, and remember the steps all at the same time. That makes dancing multitasking at its best.

Dancing is also a great stress-buster. One study found that people who tangoed for 20 minutes felt happier and had lower levels of stress hormones than people who sat on the sidelines watching.

Here's what you can expect from dancing the night away:

Ballroom dancing (e.g., tango, waltz, fox-trot)
What it does: strengthens the abs, arms, and lower back
What it burns: 190 calories per hour

Salsa and swing
What it does: increases endurance and improves coordination
What it burns: 286 calories per hour

Belly dancing and Bollywood
What it does: strengthens and defines abs, firms shoulders and arms
What it burns: 286 calories per hour

Now for the butt and thighs. This desk-ercise comes from Sara Haley, master trainer at Reebok. Scoot forward on the seat of your chair so your butt is an inch or so from the edge of the seat. Hold your legs together, making sure your knees are bent 90 degrees and your feet are together and flat on the floor. Pull your belly button in and up while you squeeze your knees and heels together to stabilize you. Then use your thigh muscles to lift your butt a few inches off the chair. Hover for 30 seconds, squeezing your butt and abs for support. Repeat a few times throughout the day. If this is too hard, try placing your feet shoulder-width apart.

Do a line dance Take advantage of some toning time while waiting in line. This move, which comes from Kristin McGee, a yoga instructor at Clay Spa in New York City, helps tone your belly and inner thighs: Stand up straight with your heels together and toes pointed slightly outward. Rise up on your toes and pull your belly button in and up, keeping your back straight. Try not to lean forward. Hold for a count of one, then slowly place your heels back on the ground. Do this 10 times— or for as long as you're waiting. The added bonus: It will distract you from whatever is holding up the line.

Don't just stand there Whenever you find yourself waiting for something—whether it's for water to boil, for an order to be ready, or for anything else—do this exercise suggested by fitness guru Kathy Smith. It will help get rid of a muffin top:

Stand with your feet hip-width apart, with your shoulders back and down. Put your left hand on your hip and your right hand behind your head. Tighten your abs, then raise your right knee to waist height and bring your right elbow down toward your knee. Try not to pop your hip out—keep the movement slow and controlled. Do this 10 times, switch sides, and do 10 times more.

Ask the EXPERT

Jennifer Cook
Senior Executive Editor, *Good Housekeeping*

Q *What is the best exercise program for someone who is obese?*

Jenny says: First, you'll want to start adding more steps to your day and more activity into your life (e.g., gardening, walking the dog). Next, focus on an aerobic activity such as walking. If that hurts your knees, try an elliptical trainer, a recumbent bicycle, or a treadmill (which can be more forgiving than pavement and therefore easier on your body). Start with a realistic goal—don't worry if it's just five minutes at a time!—and work your way up from there in increments of three to five minutes. Focus on lengthening the time you spend walking before trying to increase the intensity (like going faster or uphill). Before you start, it's a good idea to check with your doctor, especially if you have any other health conditions or risks, haven't exercised in a few months, or are over 45 (men) or 55 (women).

Q *How would you suggest I fit a workout into a full day of work, home, and family life?*

Jenny says: To get the most out of this plan, you should try to do 30 minutes of aerobic activity five times a week, strength-train a few times a week, and incorporate stretching and yoga into your schedule. It sounds like a lot, but trust me, it's doable! Nick Mastropasqua, who manages The Club at Hearst Tower and who helped develop the plan, finds that most people can carve out time in the mornings (before the rest of the household wakes up), during lunch hours, or at night (after family time has wrapped up). Which of those are workable for you? Maybe you can wake up 20 minutes earlier twice a week for strength training, take walks during lunch, and end your day with a few yoga poses before bed. Or, you could combine family and exercise time by playing a fitness video game with the kids after homework or taking family walks after dinner.

Let's Get Flexible

Stretching is like oiling your muscles and joints. It helps get blood flowing through them so you have more range of motion. And it makes everything you do, even walking, easier.

Much of what we experience as aging is actually a loss of flexibility; if you don't use your joints, tendons, and ligaments and move them through their whole range of motion, you lose mobility. Reaching becomes more difficult if your arms and shoulders are tight, while taut hamstrings can lead to lower-back pain. Keeping your body flexible is also excellent for helping you maintain your equilibrium as you age so you are less likely to lose your balance.

There's another reason to fit stretching into your day: It feels good. Stretching is like moving meditation. It gives you a little time out and helps you handle stress. Aging is, in many ways, an accumulation of stress, so anything that relieves the pressure will make you look, think, and act years younger.

How to Measure Your Flexibility

The Sit-and-Reach Test was designed by the YMCA to measure flexibility. All it requires is a yardstick; a tape measure will do, too. (Note: If you have lower-back pain, doing this might aggravate the condition.)

Remove your shoes and sit on the floor with your legs stretched out about 12 inches apart. Put the yardstick between your legs with 0 at the crotch. With your fingertips in contact with the measure, exhale as you slowly lower your head and back and stretch forward as far as possible with both hands. Note the inch mark of the farthest point your fingertips can reach. Return to the start position, take a moment to relax, and do the stretch two more times. Record your best measurement in your journal.

Redo the test weekly to measure your progress.

Get Poised for Yoga

The most profound way to help prevent the loss of equilibrium and the stiffening that come with age is to keep yourself flexible through the practice of yoga. We can read your mind already: *I can't do that. I can't even touch my toes.* You may also be thinking that you only have so much time in the day, and that the soft, flowing moves of yoga couldn't possibly help you lose weight. Maybe you're intimidated by the idea of yoga because you think it's only for waifish people who can contort themselves into human pretzels. But this is not the case at all! Yoga practice has become mainstream and can be tailored to any lifestyle. It's amazingly effective for improving flexibility in your legs and spine. And as an extra bonus, people who do yoga tend to become more mindful eaters. They are more likely to eat slowly, notice and savor the flavors of foods, recognize when portions are too large, and stop eating when they are full. One study conducted over a 10-year period found that regularly doing yoga helped prevent middle-age spread. The reason, the researchers surmised, is that yoga makes you more aware of your body and more sensitive to hunger and satiety cues. No doubt the toning that results from doing yoga helps, too.

You can learn yoga by signing up for a studio class or by buying a DVD that you can follow along with at home. All you need is some comfortable padding, like a yoga mat, and comfortable clothes. You don't even need shoes.

To show you how easy and relaxing yoga can be, here's a sample exercise for maintaining balance that is nice to do before going to bed, as it will help you relax. It's called tree pose:

Put on your pajamas and stand near the wall or a heavy piece of furniture that you can use to steady yourself as you work on your balance. Draw your hands in toward your chest with palms pressed together. Lift your right foot and press the sole and heel against the inside of your left thigh or calf, with your right knee turned outward. Breathe slowly and evenly and hold the position for 30 seconds to one minute. Switch sides and repeat.

It's the perfect move to end the day.

We like these flexibility exercises because they can be done anytime, anywhere. Work them into your day—you don't have to do them all at once—or do them as a cooldown at the end of your walk. Hold each of these stretches for 5 to 10 seconds and repeat two more times.

1. **STANDING HAMSTRING STRETCH** Stand with your legs shoulder-width apart and your knees slightly bent. Bend forward from your waist and reach your fingers toward your toes. Don't force the movement or bounce; just stretch enough to feel a comfortable tension in the backs of your legs. As you hang, let your neck and shoulders relax.

2. **STANDING CROSSOVER STRETCH** In a standing position, cross your right foot over your left. With your knees slightly bent, bend forward from your waist and reach your fingers toward your toes. Don't force the movement; just stretch far enough to feel a comfortable tension in the backs of your legs. Now cross your left foot over your right and repeat the stretch.

3. **CHEST STRETCH** Stand in an open doorway. Stretch out your arms and raise them to shoulder height, placing your hands flat on the sides of the doorframe. Lean forward until you feel a stretch through your shoulders and chest.

4. **CROSSOVER SHOULDER STRETCH** While standing or sitting, extend your right arm in front of you at shoulder height. Grasp your right elbow with your left hand and gently pull your right arm across your body, keeping it at shoulder height, until you feel a comfortable tension. Switch sides and repeat the stretch.

5. **TRICEPS STRETCH** While sitting or standing, extend your right arm over your head. Bend your right elbow so your right hand drops behind your back. Grasp your right elbow with your left hand and gently push back until you feel a good stretch in the back of your upper arm. Switch arms and repeat the stretch.

Activate Your Anti-Aging Diet Now!

1 **Add 30 minutes of movement into every day,** starting now. People who stay active throughout the day have greater success at losing weight and keeping it off. That means keeping yourself in motion as much as possible. Don't sit when you could stand; don't stand when you could pace; don't drive when you could walk or pedal. Unless you're sleeping, don't stay idle for more than an hour at a time.

2 **Start walking.** Get yourself a pedometer and a pair of walking shoes and head out the door. Work up to walking at a brisk pace with arms pumping for 30 minutes five days a week. If a half hour doesn't work into your day, aim for three 10-minute sessions. If you're up for it, jog, cycle, or hop onto an exercise machine. The idea is to get two and a half hours of heart-pumping exercise a week, even if you're just jogging in place for 10 minutes at a time.

3 **Keep your muscles strong and limber.** You're not going to achieve your goal of turning back the clock if all you can see as a result of your weight loss are jiggly muscles. Firming up with strength-training exercises and staying flexible with stretching exercises like yoga are key parts of your overall strategy for success.

For more expert anti-aging advice, get our free special report 50 Ways to Stress Less & Live Longer *at 7yearsyounger.com/stressless.*

Chapter 6

The 7 Years Younger Meal Plan

N ow for the really fun part—the food! Remember, the 7 Years Younger Meal Plan was designed with convenience and simplicity in mind.

The 3-4-5 Plan makes it easy to mix and match your meals. There's no need to count calories because we've done it all for you. All of the meals are easy to make and are designed so that you can prepare them in about 30 minutes or less. Many breakfasts and lunches can be assembled in a matter of minutes.

Every day's menu was calibrated to enrich your diet with anti-aging nutrients and is designed to fill you up so you'll never feel hungry.

Every meal includes the phytonutrient-dense fruits, vegetables, and grains that research shows promote health and help guard against age-related health problems such as high cholesterol, high blood pressure, cardiovascular disease, diabetes, and certain forms of cancer.

And here's the bonus: Specific foods in the diet were chosen because they contain nutrients that are also age erasers. Eating according to the 7 Years Younger Meal Plan will help diminish wrinkles and age spots, smooth out a rough and ruddy complexion, and give aging skin much-needed moisture. You should start to feel better, have more energy, and notice a smoother complexion and less-defined wrinkles *while you're losing weight*.

Our panelists loved the weekly meal plan and the freedom it offered to mix and match breakfasts, lunches, dinners, and snacks. "The meal plan is very simple to follow," says panelist Maria Arap. "Honestly, for me, the hardest part is picking which recipe I want to make, because I like them all. I actually look forward to planning my meals. I'm totally loving the experience."

The meal plan is not just good diet food; it's good food! Our panelists found that they could serve the recipes to the whole family rather than having to prepare separate meals for dieters and non-dieters. "The meals are really fantastic, and my two younger children, somewhat finicky eaters, have been eating basically the same dinners with no complaints," says David Sigman.

Says Lynn Bunis: "There isn't a recipe my family didn't love."

Getting Started

The 7 Years Younger Meal Plan kicks off with a Jumpstart week to get weight loss into gear. During this week, the limit for women is 1,200 calories a day over three meals. Slightly to moderately active men will get 1,450 calories a day over three meals and two 125-calorie snacks. Highly active men will get 1,575 calories, which includes the equivalent of three 125-calorie snacks. Men should look at the Jumpstart week on page 185, which includes only breakfasts, lunches, and dinners, and then turn to the snack list, starting on page 278, to choose two or three that complement the Week 1 meal plan. The best times to snack are between lunch and dinner and after the evening meal.

This first week should reveal a lot about your relationship with food—if you find yourself wanting to eat when you're bored, for example, or when you're in a social situation, or if you're following a strict schedule. It's the reason we encourage you to use a food diary and write in it every time you eat, even if you're having just one bite. Recording all your meals and how you feel during and after eating gives you insights into why you may be munching when you're not really hungry.

This first week is also the time to try out some of the strategies we recommend in Chapter 4 for helping you stay on the diet. These tactics have been scientifically proven to work, so they are all worth mastering.

Week 2 gets you on track for the rest of the program. The calorie count for women goes up to 1,450 via the addition of two 125-calorie snacks a day, one between lunch and dinner and the other between dinner and bedtime. Men will also increase their calorie counts; slightly to moderately active men will gear up to a regimen of 1,575 calories a day that includes a double portion of a 125-calorie snack and another single snack, and highly active men are bumped up to 1,700 calories a day with two double portions of 125-calorie snacks.

The Mix-and-Max Menu Plan

We designed a 3-4-5 menu plan because we found that most people eat their smallest meal in the morning (if they eat breakfast—which everyone should) and their largest meal in the evening. However, if you're someone who prefers to eat your bigger meal at lunch or breakfast, go for it. Just don't skimp on any meals or skip your snacks. The whole idea is to keep you from feeling hungry. Deprivation has no place in the 7 *Years Younger Anti-Aging Breakthrough Diet*. We don't want you to save up calories by skipping a meal or snacks so you can eat one mega-meal. This will only make you feel hungry and weaken your willpower.

As you work your way through the menus, pay special attention to the amount of food allotted at each meal. This meal plan is also a tool to teach you about portion size, the key to weight loss. All the meals are planned to supply you with the right balance of protein, carbohydrates, and fat. For example, you'll always see more fruits and vegetables at a meal than you do meat or other protein. Going from meal to meal and day to day, you will gradually become familiar with what a healthy portion size really is. You'll also learn which foods, such as whole grains, high-fiber produce, and lean protein, are the best hunger fighters—one of the most crucial lessons of the program, and one that will serve you well every time you sit down to eat.

Following the menus as designed, however, has advantages beyond letting you know how many calories there are in each meal. Each day gives you a steady infusion of health-boosting and skin-enhancing nutrients, including omega-3s, beta-carotene and other carotenoids, and vitamin C. The 7 Years Younger Meal Plan blueprint also provides:

- 3 to 6 servings of vegetables per day
- 2 to 5 servings of fruit per day
- 5 to 7 ounces of protein from animal sources (and an equivalent amount from other sources such as beans, nuts, seeds, and soy) per day
- 2 to 3 servings of low-fat dairy per day
- An average of 31 grams of fiber per day
- 2 servings of omega-3–rich fish per week

And there's tremendous variety. There are foods for every taste, from pizza, tacos, and pulled pork sandwiches to soups, stews, and turkey burgers. You'll sample foods from many different cuisines and add delicious new recipes to your repertoire. In all, nearly 100 nutritious foods guarantee that the plan will never get monotonous.

THE 7 YEARS YOUNGER MEAL PLAN

Week 1: Jumpstart

Day	Breakfast	Lunch	Dinner
1	California Breakfast Bruschetta *(page 221)*	Chipotle Lunch *(page 228)*	Big Fusilli Bowl *(page 242)*
2	Sweet Stuffed Waffle *(page 222)*	Garden Turkey Sandwich with Lemon Mayo *(page 236)*	Salmon with Peppers & Pilaf *(page 272)*
3	New York Bagel *(page 221)*	Caprese Salad *(page 228)*	Steak & Oven Fries *(page 263)*
4	Banana–Peanut Butter Smoothie *(page 223)*	Ham & Swiss *(page 229)*	Grilled Fish Tacos *(page 269)*
5	Easy Oatmeal *(page 221)*	Mediterranean Hummus "Pizza" *(page 230)*	Pulled Pork on a Bun *(page 260)*
6	Smoked-Salmon Scrambled Eggs *(page 227)*	Finger Food *(page 229)*	Turkey-Feta Burgers *(page 258)*
7	Strawberry Cereal *(page 222)*	Microwavable Pasta Meal *(page 230)*	Chicken & Veggie Stir-Fry *(page 251)*

Week 2

Day	Breakfast	Lunch	Snack 1	Dinner	Snack 2
1	New York Bagel *(page 221)*	Mediterranean Vegetarian Wrap *(page 230)*	Movie Mix *(page 279)*	Steak Sandwich with Grilled Onions *(page 264)*	Cheese Bite *(page 278)*
2	Ham & Veggie Hash *(page 225)*	Protein Plate *(page 231)*	Iced-Coffee Break *(page 279)*	Shrimp & Fresh Corn Grits *(page 274)*	Honeydew "Sundae" *(page 279)*
3	Peach Melba Yogurt *(page 222)*	Roast Beef Pockets *(page 231)*	Pistachios *(page 280)*	Chicken Lo Mein Primavera *(page 249)*	Cherries & Cheese *(page 278)*
4	Breakfast Pizza *(page 221)*	Spicy Black Bean Soup *(page 239)*	Strawberry Sipper *(page 280)*	Almond-Crusted Tilapia *(page 265)*	Out & About *(page 279)*
5	5-Minute Multigrain Cereal *(page 224)*	Shrimp Caesar Salad *(page 232)*	Pineapple Plate *(page 279)*	Spice-Rubbed Pork Tenderloin *(page 261)*	Prosciutto & Mozzarella Plate *(page 280)*
6	Berry Blast Breakfast Shake *(page 223)*	Grilled Chicken Sandwich *(page 229)*	Chips & Cheese *(page 278)*	Spaghetti with Pesto Verde *(page 244)*	Pudding Parfait *(page 280)*
7	Huevos Rancheros *(page 226)*	Sushi to Go *(page 232)*	Veggies & Dill Dip *(page 280)*	Healthy-Makeover Meatloaf *(page 254)*	Blueberry Lassi *(page 278)*

Week 3

Day	Breakfast	Lunch	Snack 1	Dinner	Snack 2
1	New York Bagel *(page 221)*	Grilled Mozzarella & Tomato Soup *(page 229)*	PB & J-Inspired Yogurt *(page 279)*	Seared Salmon with Sweet Potatoes *(page 274)*	Ricotta-Fig Toasts *(page 280)*
2	Peach Melba Yogurt *(page 222)*	Ham & Swiss *(page 229)*	Hummus & Veggie Strips *(page 279)*	Basil-Orange Chicken with Couscous *(page 247)*	Chips & Cheese *(page 278)*
3	Easy Oatmeal *(page 221)*	Cold Peanut Noodles with Chicken *(page 228)*	Iced-Coffee Break *(page 279)*	Two-Cheese Pita Pizzas with Broccoli & Tomato *(page 245)*	Cantaloupe Boat *(page 278)*
4	Sunrise Soft Taco *(page 222)*	Microwavable Pasta Meal *(page 230)*	Citrus Snack *(page 278)*	Chicken Parm Stacks *(page 250)*	Out & About *(page 279)*
5	Breakfast to Go *(page 221)*	Chicken Caesar Pitas *(page 234)*	Strawberry Bagel Thin *(page 280)*	Niçoise Salad *(page 270)*	Cocoa Fix *(page 278)*
6	Banana-Peanut Butter Smoothie *(page 223)*	Subway Sandwich & Soup *(page 232)*	Cherries & Cheese *(page 278)*	Pomegranate-Glazed Salmon *(page 271)*	Edamame Munchie *(page 278)*
7	Breakfast Pizza *(page 221)*	Asian Chicken Salad *(page 233)*	Honeydew "Sundae" *(page 279)*	Beef Ragu *(page 262)*	Fruit & Grain Bar *(page 279)*

Ask the EXPERT

Samantha B. Cassetty, M.S., R.D.
Nutrition Director, GHRI

Q *I've been cutting back on salt—and I miss it! Any advice?*

Samantha says: Give it some time. Studies show that it can take your taste buds as little as six to eight weeks to adjust to a lower-sodium diet, at which point the food you previously enjoyed will taste too salty. Also note that up to three-quarters of the salt in your diet comes from packaged foods, not the shaker. Since the 7 Years Younger Meal Plan recipes use some ingredient shortcuts (canned beans, for example, instead of dried ones), a few meals are somewhat high in sodium. Not to worry, though: Averaged out over the course of the day, sodium levels on the plan remain well within healthy limits.

Q *I eat fish and dairy, but I don't eat any meat or poultry. What's your advice for following the 7 Years Younger Anti-Aging Breakthrough Diet?*

Samantha says: If you're a fish-eating vegetarian (technically, a pescatarian), you'll create your 3-4-5 program using the wide variety of seafood dishes and already-meatless meals on the 7 Years Younger Meal Plan. Strawberry Cereal (page 222), Shrimp Caesar Salad (page 232), and Two-Cheese Pita Pizzas with Broccoli & Tomato (page 245) are some of the meals you can enjoy.

If fish isn't on your menu, you'll rely on the plan's meat-free selections, but you can also call on your inner foodie to get creative with swaps—for example, substituting beans for fish in our Grilled Fish Tacos (page 269), using tofu instead of shrimp in our Soba Noodle Bowl with Shrimp & Snow Peas (page 276), or simply omitting the small amount of chicken in the Chicken Lo Mein Primavera (page 249). See the chart at right for help with meatless protein swaps.

The lunch menu, with an assortment of vegetarian meals, can also be used for dinner and will allow you an extra snack on days you make this swap. Or, take a look at our frozen entrée options on page 76–77; most of them will work for you. Since a meal plan lacking in protein can leave you hungry, make sure you're getting enough protein-rich beans, nuts, cheese, and Greek yogurt at meals and snacks.

Vegetarian Protein Picks

Beans, nuts, and soy are great, protein-packed alternatives to meat. When making substitutions in meals, consider these options. Each has roughly the same calories as 3 ounces of cooked chicken breast (140).

Pick a Protein (Serving Size)	Calories
Sunflower seeds (½ cup)	134
Fat-free refried beans (⅔ cup)	137
Almonds (20 nuts)	138
Soy nuts (⅓ cup)	138
Kidney beans (⅔ cup)	139
Chickpeas (⅔ cup)	139
Peanut butter (smooth or chunky) (1½ Tbsp.)	141
Cashew butter (1½ Tbsp.)	141
Edamame (¾ cup)	143
Firm tofu (6 oz.)	143
Pumpkin seeds (½ cup)	143
Macadamia nuts (8 nuts)	144
Walnuts (11 halves)	144
Black beans (⅔ cup)	144
Cashews (16 nuts)	145
Peanuts (25 nuts)	146
Almond butter (1½ Tbsp.)	147
Lentils (⅔ cup cooked lentils)	152

Week 4

Day	Breakfast	Lunch	Snack 1	Dinner	Snack 2
1	Huevos Rancheros (page 226)	Open-Face Jarlsberg Sandwich with Greens (page 237)	Blueberry Lassi (page 278)	Orange Pork & Asparagus Stir-Fry (page 259)	Pistachios (page 280)
2	Easy Oatmeal (page 221)	Chinese Rice Bowl (page 228)	Prosciutto & Mozzarella Plate (page 280)	Lemon-Mint Chicken Cutlets on Watercress (page 255)	Cheese Bite (page 278)
3	Strawberry Cereal (page 222)	Chipotle Lunch (page 228)	Hummus & Veggie Strips (page 279)	Garden-Vegetable Omelet (page 243)	Pudding Parfait (page 280)
4	Sweet Stuffed Waffle (page 222)	Greek Feast (page 229)	Iced-Coffee Break (page 279)	Crispy Fish Sandwiches (page 267)	Movie Mix (page 279)
5	Smoked-Salmon Scrambled Eggs (page 227)	Mexican Chicken Salad (page 230)	Pineapple Plate (page 279)	Ziti with Peas, Grape Tomatoes & Ricotta (page 246)	Chips & Cheese (page 278)
6	Grab & Go (page 221)	Grilled Mozzarella & Tomato Soup (page 229)	Veggies & Dill Dip (page 280)	Chicken & Veggie Stir-Fry (page 251)	Ricotta-Fig Toasts (page 280)
7	California Breakfast Bruschetta (page 221)	Jambalaya (page 230)	Yogurt Sundae (page 280)	Fresh Salmon Burgers with Capers and Dill (page 268)	Cantaloupe Boat (page 278)

Week 5

Day	Breakfast	Lunch	Snack 1	Dinner	Snack 2
1	Sunrise Soft Taco (page 222)	Finger Food (page 229)	Honeydew "Sundae" (page 279)	Spice-Rubbed Pork Tenderloin (page 261)	Cherries & Cheese (page 278)
2	Breakfast to Go (page 221)	Garden Turkey Sandwich with Lemon Mayo (page 236)	Strawberry Bagel Thin (page 280)	Healthy-Makeover Meatloaf (page 254)	Cocoa Fix (page 278)
3	Breakfast Pizza (page 221)	Mexican Meal in Minutes (page 230)	Hummus & Veggie Strips (page 279)	Chicken with Berry Sauce (page 248)	Prosciutto & Mozzarella Plate (page 280)
4	New York Bagel (page 221)	Roast Beef Chef's Salad (page 231)	PB & J- Inspired Yogurt (page 279)	Steamed Scrod Fillet Dinner (page 277)	Out & About (page 279)
5	Banana-Peanut Butter Smoothie (page 223)	Creole Chicken Frankfurter Meal (page 228)	Chips & Cheese (page 278)	Curried Chicken Salad (page 252)	Edamame Munchie (page 278)
6	Easy Oatmeal (page 221)	Sandwich & Slaw (page 232)	Citrus Snack (page 278)	Soba Noodle Bowl with Shrimp & Snow Peas (page 276)	Movie Mix (page 279)
7	Ham & Veggie Hash (page 225)	Easy Cobb Salad (page 235)	Iced-Coffee Break (page 279)	Fajitas Two Ways (page 253)	Pudding Parfait (page 280)

Week 6

Day	Breakfast	Lunch	Snack 1	Dinner	Snack 2
1	Sweet Stuffed Waffle (page 222)	Peanut Butter & Apple Sandwich (page 231)	Pistachios (page 281)	Chipotle-Orange-Glazed Salmon (page 266)	Cheese Bite (page 278)
2	New York Bagel (page 221)	Spinach & Nectarine Salad (page 240)	Iced-Coffee Break (page 279)	Steak & Oven Fries (page 263)	Fruit & Grain Bar (page 279)
3	Breakfast to Go (page 221)	Veggie Burger (page 232)	Cantaloupe Boat (page 278)	Lemon-Oregano Chicken Cutlets with Mint Zucchini (page 256)	Strawberry Sipper (page 280)
4	Huevos Rancheros (page 226)	Tuna & Cannellini Bean Salad (page 241)	Cherries & Cheese (page 278)	Turkey-Escarole Soup (page 257)	Veggies & Dill Dip (page 280)
5	Berry Blast Breakfast Shake (page 223)	Creole Chicken Frankfurter Meal (page 228)	Ricotta-Fig Toasts (page 280)	Big Fusilli Bowl (page 242)	Prosciutto & Mozzarella Plate (page 280)
6	5-Minute Multigrain Cereal (page 224)	Subway Sandwich & Soup (page 232)	Citrus Snack (page 278)	Scallop & Cherry Tomato Skewers (page 273)	Out & About (page 279)
7	Grab & Go (page 221)	No-Cook Bean Burrito (page 231)	Cocoa Fix (page 278)	Chicken Parm Stacks (page 250)	Yogurt Sundae (page 280)

Week 7

Day	Breakfast	Lunch	Snack 1	Dinner	Snack 2
1	Breakfast Pizza (page 221)	Cheesy Chili (page 228)	Movie Mix (page 279)	Healthy-Makeover Meatloaf (page 254)	Pineapple Plate (page 279)
2	Ham & Veggie Hash (page 225)	Sushi to Go (page 232)	PB & J-Inspired Yogurt (page 279)	Ziti with Peas, Grape Tomatoes & Ricotta (page 246)	Cheese Bite (page 278)
3	Banana-Peanut Butter Smoothie (page 223)	Mexican Meal in Minutes (page 230)	Strawberry Bagel Thin (page 280)	Turkey-Feta Burgers (page 258)	Pudding Parfait (page 280)
4	Strawberry Cereal (page 222)	Asian Chicken Salad (page 233)	Iced-Coffee Break (page 279)	Almond-Crusted Tilapia (page 265)	Hummus & Veggie Strips (page 279)
5	California Breakfast Bruschetta (page 221)	Mediterranean Hummus "Pizza" (page 230)	Blueberry Lassi (page 278)	Chicken & Veggie Stir-Fry (page 251)	Chips & Cheese (page 278)
6	Sweet Stuffed Waffle (page 222)	Southwest Chicken Wraps (page 238)	Cantaloupe Boat (page 278)	Spice-Rubbed Pork Tenderloin (page 261)	Cocoa Fix (page 278)
7	Peach Melba Yogurt (page 222)	Finger Food (page 229)	Edamame Munchie (page 278)	Seared Salmon with Sweet Potatoes (page 274)	Prosciutto & Mozzarella Plate (page 280)

Ask the EXPERT

Samantha B. Cassetty, M.S., R.D.
Nutrition Director, GHRI

Q *I'm a chip-oholic. Which ones are best to snack on? There are so many brands out there.*

Samantha says: Chips can be part of your 7 Years Younger eating plan as long as you choose ones that supply anti-aging nutrients. My favorite munchies are SunChips and Food Should Taste Good Multigrain Chips because both are chock-full of whole grains and have 3 grams of appetite-thwarting fiber. I'm also wild about Terra Sweet Potato Chips (also with 3 grams of fiber), made from just sweet potatoes and oil. Next best are tortilla chips made with whole corn (such as regular or baked Tostitos). Also, while it's not chips, my son and I can't resist air-popped popcorn: It's 100% whole-grain and is loaded with healthy plant compounds, but has just 30 calories per cup.

One more bit of advice: Take a look at the calories and portion sizes on chip bags and note how we use chips on the plan. You'll see that a normal portion is above our 125-calorie snack limit, and since chips lack protein, they're not the best snack option on their own. For maximum hunger-fighting benefits, we've paired a smaller number of them with a protein (such as 5 Food Should Taste Good chips with a cheese stick), so follow our example whenever you snack on chips.

Q *I'm the kind of person who really wants a cookie (or two!) before bed. Can any of the options out there work as an after-dinner snack?*

Samantha says: I understand your predicament, so I dug up a few options that are made predominantly with whole grains, have a reasonable amount of sugar, and clock in at no more than 130 calories per serving. Here are my picks:

- 100% Whole Grain Fig Newtons (2 cookies)
- Back to Nature Apple Cinnamon Oat Grahams (2 full sheets), Golden Honey Oat Grahams (2 full sheets), or Crispy Oatmeal Cookies (2 cookies)
- Barbara's Bakery Snackimals in Wheat Free Oatmeal (about 10 cookies)
- Kashi Cookies (1 cookie) in Chocolate Almond Butter, Oatmeal Raisin Flax, or Oatmeal Dark Chocolate
- Willamette Valley Granola Company Granola Chips (about 20 chips) in Butter Pecan, Vanilla Bean, and Honey Nut

Now the "gotchas": The 7 Years Younger Meal Plan is designed to dial down your sweet tooth and help keep you looking and feeling young, so cookies aren't on the daily menu. It's OK to substitute one of these treats for a snack once per week, but they won't be as satisfying as the snacks on our meal plan, because they lack protein. Also, no going back for seconds!

Chapter 7

Take Your Diet to Dinner

There is no situation in which your good dieting intentions are put to the test more than when you're dining out. Though the *7 Years Younger Anti-Aging Breakthrough Diet* is designed around a menu plan that calls mainly for eat-at-home meals, there is no need for restaurant meals to be off-limits. And we know what a big part of your life eating out probably is: One survey found that the average American dines away from home five times a week. If that sounds like you, you need to be mindful about what you order and how much you consume, especially if eating out is a part of your daily life rather than a treat. Dining out most definitely can be a part of your new get-thin-and-stay-thin life, provided you recognize the pitfalls and learn how to avoid them. And if you're the kind of person who dines out more than you eat in, you should be fine as long as you order meals that fit within the *7 Years Younger Anti-Aging Breakthrough Diet* guidelines.

How Restaurants Fool You

The problem with dining out is the temptation to overindulge, something that restaurants make all too easy. One study found that restaurant meals typically contain 60% more calories than meals prepared at home. And those calories are not all that easy to spot; even experts can be fooled. When a New York University researcher asked 200 dietitians to estimate the calorie counts of four popular restaurant dishes, they lowballed them by a whopping 200 to 700 calories—that can be almost half your daily calories on the 7 *Years Younger Anti-Aging Breakthrough Diet*! When the California Center for Public Health Advocacy asked 523 people to name the healthiest options at popular restaurants, 68% didn't get a single answer right.

The main reason? Restaurant portions can be B–I-G. In many restaurants, pasta portions that typically would feed a family of four are served to a single diner. You'd think dining out would be a lot easier on the waist-

The Slice Is Right

We love pizza; you love pizza; your family loves pizza. So how do you dine out on pizza, which is so notoriously full of calories, while trying to lose weight? By forgoing the extras—like high-calorie and high-fat sausage, pepperoni, and meatballs—that help pile on pounds. Instead, pile on the veggies—mushrooms, bell peppers, fresh tomatoes, eggplant, and more. They offer minimal calories and virtually no fat. Here's an example of how easy it is to slice back: At Pizza Hut, you could save 150 calories per slice simply by passing on the Meat Lover's Pizza and going for the Veggie Lover's Pizza with the Thin 'N Crispy crust.

For the most slimming slices, go for the thinnest possible crust and ask the pizzeria to use half the usual amount of cheese. Consider ordering a pie with no cheese and sprinkling the top with Parmesan instead. Another great idea is to implement a one-slice limit and fill up on salad.

line now that a federal mandate requires chain restaurants with 20 or more locations to make public their nutritional facts on all menu items. These eateries are located on major roads in urban areas all across America, and throngs of people frequent them almost daily. The mandatory menu nutritional analysis is an idea the public is embracing: Surveys indicate that more than a third of restaurant patrons go online to look up the calorie counts of menu items before they head out to eat. But even here, appearances can be deceiving. The government mandates that calorie counts must be posted, but nobody is regulating restaurants' portion sizes.

So be forewarned: When checking out nutritional stats at your favorite chains, make sure to check out the calories and the serving size. Though the calorie count may be posted somewhere in the restaurant, you probably won't find it on the menu next to the dish's description. When you know you're going out to eat—and especially if you are the kind of person who eats out more often than you cook at home—do your homework ahead of time so you won't get caught off guard: Check websites, which often list calorie counts (although you may need to spend a few minutes tracking down the info). Consider restaurant meals that are approved on the plan and assemble a similar meal at your local eatery, double up on veggies, and lighten up on the grains.

Dining Out Smartly

Our panel of dieters discovered dining out was not nearly as hard as they'd thought it would be thanks to the following trusty tips, and almost everyone had several occasions to dine out during their seven-week test run. To arm yourself against unwanted calories and fat, here's what to do before crossing a restaurant threshold:

Do your homework Many restaurants post their menus online, something you should check out before making a reservation. They generally are easy to find; just search for the restaurant's name followed by "nutri-

Test Your Calorie IQ

Getting familiar with calories is key to losing weight, but restaurant menus don't make it easy. Can you pick the low-calorie choice at these eight chain eateries?

Restaurant	A	B
Applebee's	French Onion Soup Bowl	Oriental Grilled Chicken Salad
Outback Steakhouse	9-oz. Victoria's Filet of Beef	Alice Springs Chicken
Panera Bread	Asiago Roast Beef Sandwich	Sierra Turkey Sandwich
Quiznos	Regular Honey Bourbon Chicken Sandwich	Regular Veggie Guacamole Sandwich
Red Lobster	Bowl of Manhattan Clam Chowder	Bowl of Seafood Gumbo
Ruby Tuesday	Avocado Turkey Burger	Ribs and Louisiana Fried Shrimp
Subway	6-Inch Roast Beef Sandwich	6-Inch Tuna Sandwich
Taco Bell	Beef Burrito Supreme	Fiesta Chicken Taco Salad

If you mostly picked A, give yourself a gold star. If you're like a lot of people, though, you probably went for B in many cases. That could end up costing you 150 to 800 calories, depending on the meal. If you actually ate those choices, it would cost you 3,253 calories, or nearly a pound! A salad might seem like the

tional analysis" or "nutritional information," and the menu for your restaurant should pop up. Take the time to read it, not just scan it, and decide ahead of time what you'll order.

Choose by food, not by restaurant Before you head out to a restaurant, go to healthydiningfinder.com, which recommends menu items that meet a set of criteria determined by a team of nutritionists and dietitians. The obvious choice, but Applebee's Oriental Grilled Chicken Salad packs nearly a day's worth of calories on top of a pile of nearly calorie-free greens—choosing the cheesy soup actually saves an astounding 920 calories. The lesson of this exercise: Check out calorie counts online before dining out. For the record, here's how the choices tab out:

Applebee's: French Onion Soup Bowl: 370 calories; Oriental Grilled Chicken Salad: 1,290 calories. *Savings: 920 calories*

Outback Steakhouse: Victoria's Filet of Beef: 338 calories; Alice Springs Chicken: 1,139 calories (with fries). *Savings: 801 calories*

Panera Bread: Asiago Roast Beef Sandwich: 710 calories; Sierra Turkey Sandwich: 920 calories. *Savings: 210 calories*

Quiznos: Honey Bourbon Chicken Sandwich: 530 calories; Veggie Guacamole Sandwich: 760 calories. *Savings: 230 calories*

Red Lobster: Manhattan Clam Chowder: 160 calories; Seafood Gumbo: 470 calories. *Savings: 310 calories*

Ruby Tuesday: Avocado Turkey Burger: 908 calories; Ribs and Louisiana Fried Shrimp: 1,060 calories. *Savings: 152 calories*

Subway: Roast Beef Sandwich: 320 calories; Tuna Sandwich: 470 calories. *Savings: 150 calories*

Taco Bell: Beef Burrito Supreme: 420 calories; Fiesta Chicken Taco Salad: 730 calories. *Savings: 310 calories*

site is partially funded by the Centers for Disease Control and Prevention. Approximately 30,000 chain and independent establishments nationwide are listed in its database. All you have to do is go to the website and type in your zip code: The names of the participating restaurants in your area will come up along with the number of and a list of healthy items offered on their menus.

Ask the EXPERT

Samantha B. Cassetty, M.S., R.D.
Nutrition Director, GHRI

Q *I have a vacation coming up. Can you give me tips for staying on track while I'm away?*

Samantha says: Vacation is a time to focus on maintaining your weight loss rather than shedding extra pounds. Chances are you'll be eating out more than usual, so think about what your *7 Years Younger Anti-Aging Breakthrough Diet* menu looks like and follow it in spirit. Breakfast might be fruit and yogurt or a veggie omelet with a slice of whole wheat toast; lunch could be a big salad topped with grilled chicken or an open-face sandwich; dinner could include seafood or a lean cut of pork or steak along with plenty of veggies. Avoid pasta and grain-based entrées, since restaurants tend to serve gigantic portions.

Tempting as it might be, I'd also pass on a restaurant dessert. The servings tend to be humongous, and thus their calorie counts are often way over the top (1,000-plus calories in some cases!). If you can't resist an evening sweet, stop at a chocolate shop and buy one truffle or head to a pastry place and have a small cookie.

Finally, I'd like to help you recast your thinking about dining out, whether on vacation or in your hometown. Consider a meal away from home a chance to relax while someone else is doing the cooking and the cleaning. That makes the *experience* a treat—not just the meal.

One last bit of vacation advice: Pack some comfortable shoes and walk, walk, walk!

Q *Can I have a glass of wine or a bottle of beer on the plan?*

Samantha says: Yes! And spirits, too, if that's what you're in the mood for. Just stick to one a day, steer clear of high-cal mixers like syrups, juices, and sodas (that goes for frozen drinks, too), and have your drink in place of a snack. In maintenance mode, men can have two drinks a day, but women still need to stop at one. This amount of alcohol is linked to anti-aging perks, like a lower risk of heart disease, stroke, and diabetes. More than that, however, is tied to health problems, which is why it's important to stick to this limit. It's also not a good idea to "save" your daily drink for girls' (or guys') night out, since that type of drinking can also lead to health troubles.

Q *I don't want to do all that cooking. What are my options? Which types of restaurant cuisines work best with the 7 Years Younger style of eating?*

Samantha says: I hear you! On the *7 Years Younger Anti-Aging Breakthrough Diet*, there are plenty of ways to dine on nights when you want to give your pots and pans a rest. On pages 212–214, you'll find a long list of suggested orders from popular national chain restaurants, all of which fit within the calorie framework of the 7 Years Younger Meal Plan. Or you can swap in a lunch for a dinner, since the lunches tend to involve less time in the kitchen. On days when you do, feel free to have an extra snack to make up the calorie difference. Also, on pages 281–282 you'll find seven easy ways to transform a store-bought rotisserie chicken into a flavorful meal—with just five ingredients and hardly any chopping required!

Q *I know I shouldn't skip any meals, but can I eat fewer calories during the week so I can splurge on the weekend?*

Samantha says: In general, no. Here's why: Unlike many diets that treat calories like a savings account (you have a certain number to spend, and it's up to you how and when to spend them), the 7 Years Younger Meal Plan emphasizes the quality of the calories (foods that fill you up) and the pattern of eating (three meals, two snacks), which keeps blood sugar levels steady. Together, these two tactics quash hunger so you can lose weight without feeling deprived.

There is one exception, though. If you have a special event coming up—like a graduation party or anniversary dinner—then a scaling-back approach is a smart strategy. I'd suggest having slightly smaller portions throughout the week or having lunches for dinner (without the extra snack). Come party time, take a "Worth it or not?" approach to the menu. I'm a donut lover, so I never pass up homemade versions at a Mother's Day brunch, for example, but I always say no to the standard coffee shop varieties that show up after each of my son's Little League games.

Get cozy with your faves If, like most people, you tend to frequent the same spots over and over again, get familiar with the menu and the manager or your favorite server at each. Ask questions about individual ingredients you want to avoid, like "Does the soup have cream?" Don't hesitate to make special requests, such as for whole wheat pasta or brown rice, or ask if the chef will pan-fry instead of deep-fry or bake instead of sauté in order to save you calories. Most chefs are happy to accommodate such requests, especially when it comes to their regular customers.

Be informed when ordering Generally speaking, grilled chicken, fish, or even a lean cut of beef such as sirloin or tenderloin is a good bet. If something is topped with a sauce, ask if it contains cream or oil. If so, pass on the item or ask for it on the side. Skip the potato—even an unadorned baked one can be a giant—and request a second veggie instead. Choose a vinaigrette salad dressing and order it on the side. Offer up a polite "No, thank you" to the bread basket.

Words like "battered" or "crispy" usually mean an item is fried, while "au gratin," "creamed," and "scalloped" indicate that it's loaded with cream or cheese or both. Terms such as "grilled," "baked," "broiled," and "roasted" tend to indicate healthier and lower-calorie options.

Dieter's Top Tip

Don't Go to Dinner Hungry

Neil Fredman set himself up for success with this simple pre-mealtime strategy: To make sure his hunger didn't get the best of him, he got in the habit of eating an apple about a half hour before his evening meal. "That time lapse makes a difference," he says. "I didn't sit down for dinner feeling famished."

Because it is so hard to gauge a restaurant menu item's calories, it is best to avoid grains and rice-based dishes, as they probably contain too much butter, oil, or cream. Say "No, thank you" when the waiter wants to bring the dessert menu. Restaurant desserts tend to be oversize, so the calories are really over the top. But if you wait until you get home to have a small piece of dark chocolate, you can still end your meal on a sweet note without breaking the caloric bank.

Start with soup Soup does more than help you warm up on a cold day: It helps you eat less. Studies at Pennsylvania State University have found that people who start with soup eat less of their entrées, for a calorie savings of an amazing 10%. It's a great strategy when dining out. However, be careful how you order, as soup can be deceptively high in calories. Think clear or brothy soups, like miso or Manhattan clam chowder—milk- and cream-based soups, such as New England clam chowder and cream of broccoli, and soups with the word "cheese" associated with them, are too high in calories to be helpful.

These are some examples of smart picks when dining out:

- Panera Bread Bistro French Onion Soup without cheese and croutons, 190 calories per cup
- P.F. Chang's Egg Drop Soup, 7 ounces, 60 calories
- Olive Garden Minestrone, 8 ounces, 100 calories
- Qdoba Tortilla Soup, 6 ounces, 65 calories
- Quiznos Chicken Noodle Soup, 6 ounces, plus two crackers, 140 calories

Listen to your stomach Because restaurant portions are typically oversize, it is especially important to pay attention to what your stomach is telling you when you're dining out. As soon as you start to feel full, put down your fork, spoon, or sandwich and wait it out for a few minutes. Repeat this mantra to yourself: *Clean plates are not required.* You don't want to eat to the point of discomfort. The idea is to feel satisfied, not stuffed.

The Salad Bar "Take 10"

The innocent salad bar has descended from the realm of diet delight to that of diet disaster—as in, do we really need potatoes, salami slivers, and crispy wonton wedges on our greens? The real calorie bomb, though, is usually found in the ladle of dressing it takes to top the mile-high mound of all-you-can-eat salad mix-ins.

But this is not to say you should avoid the salad bar. After all, what better place is there to find a full day's worth of fruits and vegetables at just one meal? The key is to navigate it to your weight-loss advantage while still giving your taste buds a treat. We recommend that you grab a plate, count off the salad bar 10 below, and ignore the rest. Here's how to handpick a lunch salad meal that adds up to roughly 400 calories:

1 **Leafy greens** The greener, the better—and the tastier. Iceberg is appropriately named because it tastes like solid water and needs a bath in dressing to give it a kick. Healthier greens such as romaine, arugula, spinach, mesclun, watercress, and mustard greens, just to name a few, are full of flavor on their own.
How much? Go for it. The sky's the limit.
Calories? Let's call these a freebie.

2 **Beans** Loaded with protein, fiber, and nutrients, full-of-flavor beans make you feel fuller faster and help you stay satisfied longer. Garbanzo beans and kidney beans are the kinds typically found at salad bars.
How much? Around 2 tablespoons
Calories? About 40

3 **Fresh raw veggies** Think of the color code and go for the unprocessed offerings—broccoli, carrots, green beans, red cabbage, tomatoes, peppers, etc. Just steer clear of the already doctored-up versions of potato salad, coleslaw, and more.
How much? Limit starchy veggies, such as corn and potatoes, which tend to be high in calories, to a quarter-cup. Otherwise, the sky's the limit.
Calories? About 30

4 **Fresh fruit** When the fruit is fresh and not packed in syrup, it will give your salad a nice tang and your body an infusion of phytochemicals, vitamins, minerals, and fiber. Dried fruits, which are also typical at a salad bar, are

good, too, although you should be mindful of how much you're taking.

How much? Around ½ cup fresh or 2 tablespoons dried

Calories? About 40

5 **Nuts and seeds** Their yummy crunch is wholesomely packed with protein and nutrients.

How much? They're high in calories, but it only takes a little to boost the nutrition and add flavor. Keep it to 1 tablespoon.

Calories? Around 45

6 **Cheese** You don't need to skip this taste treat; just keep it in check. You'll get the most flavor from crumbled feta or grated Parmesan, both popular salad-bar features.

How much? About 1 tablespoon

Calories? Around 25

7 **Olives** A decadent treat that offers a mouthful of flavor—a little goes a long way—from super-healthy monounsaturated fat.

How much? Around 2 tablespoons sliced or 3 to 4 whole olives

Calories? About 30

8 **Hard-boiled eggs** Lots of protein (6 grams per egg) can help make your salad a satisfying complete meal.

How much? Around 2 tablespoons chopped, or half an egg

Calories? About 35

9 **Grilled skinless chicken breast** A low-calorie, protein-rich option to pair with your greens. It also helps you stay fuller longer.

How much? Around ¼ cup shredded or cubed

Calories? About 60

10 **Light dressing** Don't pick up that ladle! It will add hundreds of calories to your salad. Scan the dressings and look for the lightest among the selections. The word to look for is "vinaigrette." Bring your spoon from your table setup to the salad bar with you and use it to drizzle your dressing over the top.

How much? Aim for 2 tablespoons. If you're using a teaspoon from your place setting, that would be 6 spoonfuls.

Calories? Around 60

Ask the EXPERT

Samantha B. Cassetty, M.S., R.D.
Nutrition Director, GHRI

Q *What's your advice for getting through the holidays without putting on the pounds—or making too many sacrifices?*

Samantha says: Routines tend to get sidelined during the holidays, so I suggest trying to maintain your weight loss rather than focusing on losing more. Think ahead and determine what your social calendar looks like: Do you have parties three nights this week? Then plan to grocery-shop ahead of schedule so you can treat yourself to 7 Years Younger Meal Plan dinners the other evenings. The goal is to follow the plan as much as possible so you can indulge a little on your off nights. But don't go crazy! Decide on one splurge—a few hors d'oeuvres or a small helping of dessert (not both)—and fill up on crudités, salad, and lean protein. (See the chart at right for a look at how party fare adds up—and advice on how to make better picks.)

Remember to keep track of liquid calories from Champagne, wine, eggnog, and other favorite holiday drinks. Alcohol, while allowed on the *7 Years Younger Anti-Aging Breakthrough Diet*, can derail your efforts if you overdo it, since it not only adds calories, but also weakens your willpower—especially problematic in a party setting with calorie traps (fried shrimp! baked Brie!) everywhere you turn.

Exercise also deserves a mention, since it's the first thing one tends to drop from a crowded to-do list. Make an attempt to wear your pedometer as often as possible—say, for a lap around the office, grocery store, or mall—to boost your activity levels.

Finally, I also suggest that you try visualization techniques, which are very effective with athletes, to imagine what it will look like as you carry out this plan (pages 138–140 explain how)—doing so will help firm up your resolve. It's also a good idea to bring to mind all the nonfood things that make the holidays special; for me, they're a chance to reconnect with my family and dearest friends, reflect on my spirituality, and enjoy seasonal decorations.

Party On!

Holiday food isn't exactly diet fare, but some picks won't weigh you down as much as others. Here's a look at some popular party options as well as some lighter, but equally festive, alternatives.

Party Pass	Cal.	Party Pick	Cal.	Cal. Saved
Pecan pie	503	Pumpkin pie	316	187
Fruitcake	205	Angel food cake	140	65
Eggnog	440	Light eggnog	80	360
Mulled wine	200	Spiced cider with rum	150	50
Creamy scalloped potatoes	295	Roasted potatoes	125	170
5 pigs in blankets	300	5 jumbo shrimp	220	80
1 handful of potato chips with 2 Tbsp. French onion dip	220	1 handful of buttered popcorn	40	180
1 handful of peanuts	165	1 handful of mini pretzels	50	115
3 cheese straws	130	1 handful of Cheddar Goldfish	50	80
6 bacon-wrapped dates	450	6 prosciutto-wrapped asparagus spears	168	282

Avoid buffets All-you-can-eat buffets are not only an invitation to gorge, but also a trap. That's what researchers at Cornell University's Food and Brand Lab found when they watched the way 213 diners approached all-you-can-eat Chinese-food buffets. They recognized that patrons who were thin and those who were heavy had different behavior patterns. The overweight people chose larger plates over smaller ones, dug right in at the start of the buffet rather than scanning the offerings, and sat facing the buffet table, an enticement to return. So keep that in mind next time you find yourself near a buffet: Grab a smaller plate, cruise through all the offerings before you start filling up, and do your best not to look at the buffet once you sit back down. Also remember: Even though it's all-you-can-eat, you'll probably end up regretting it if you eat more than you *should* eat. If you find buffets too hard to resist, just avoid them and opt for ordering off the menu instead.

Don't conserve calories for a big event. Skimping on meals or, even worse, skipping them to save calories for a dining-out splurge is a common, but misguided, strategy. At the end of the day, you'll wind up eating more calories than you would have if you had eaten two normal meals. "Reserving" calories will mean that you'll arrive at the restaurant famished, with your guard down. Rather than order what your rational mind wants, your irrational mind will push you to order a calorie bomb. Why tempt yourself?

Substitute to save Make strategic choices when you're dining out so you'll enjoy your meal without going overboard. If breakfast at the diner is just not the same without bacon, then order it with poached eggs instead of fried ones and skip the home fries. If the french fries at your favorite bistro are "to die for," then order fish instead of steak and share fries with the table. There is no reason to forgo dessert during your anniversary celebration, but share one instead of ordering two.

Practice damage control In the real world of dining out, making hard choices is not always possible. So before you walk into a situation that will likely involve a few indulgences, figure out a plan for how you're going to neutralize the damage. Visualize walking into the restaurant, sitting down, and ordering something healthy, like salmon and veggies. Cut back on your snacks through the next few mealtimes, and kick up your activity level. Do whatever is necessary so the memory of the meal will reside in your mind and not on your hips.

Eating Out Made Easy

When you want to set your cutting board aside and dine out, there are plenty of options that closely adhere to the age-defying guidelines of the 7 Years Younger Meal Plan. Though restaurant meals are notoriously oversize and high in sodium and it's not always possible to find whole grains on the menu, that doesn't mean there aren't still plenty of options for you. Eating out is a part of a balanced and enjoyable life, and it's fine to occasionally bend the rules. Turn the page to find your healthiest meal options from some of America's favorite eateries.

Healthier Lunch Options

Restaurant	Meal	Calories
Arby's	Turkey Classic Roaster Sandwich, Chopped Side Salad with Light Italian dressing, Apple Slices (from the Value Menu)	405
Arby's	Classic Roast Beef Sandwich, Apple Slices (from the Value Menu)	395
KFC	Grilled Chicken Breast with Honey BBQ Dipping Sauce, Individual Sides of Whole Kernel Corn and Green Beans	385
KFC	Grilled Drumstick and Grilled Thigh with Honey BBQ Dipping Sauce, Individual Sides of Whole Kernel Corn and Green Beans	395
McDonald's	Premium Bacon Ranch Salad with Grilled Chicken Fillet and Newman's Own Low Fat Balsamic Vinaigrette, Medium Nonfat Latte	400
Moe's Southwest Grill	Burrito Bowl with Chicken, Steak, Ground Beef, or Tofu (no rice)*	404-424
Moe's Southwest Grill	Burrito Bowl with Fish*	379
Olive Garden	Pasta e Fagioli Soup, Venetian Apricot Chicken (lunch portion)	420
Olive Garden	Minestrone Soup, Linguine Alla Marinara (lunch portion)	410
Panera Bread	All Natural Low Fat Chicken Noodle Soup (1 cup), half of a Smoked Ham & Swiss on Rye sandwich (from the You Pick Two menu)	370
Panera Bread	Low Fat Garden Vegetable with Pesto Soup (1 cup), half of a Chicken Cobb with Avocado Salad (from the You Pick Two menu)	390
Panera Bread	Half Caesar Salad, half of a Smoked Turkey Breast sandwich on Country Bread (from the You Pick Two menu)	370
Starbucks	Bistro Box Protein Plate	380
Starbucks	Chipotle Chicken Wrap, Seasonal Harvest Fruit Blend	380

*Order with black beans, shredded lettuce, southwestern slaw, grilled 'shrooms, cucumbers, tomatoes, onions, pico de gallo, and cilantro

Restaurant	Meal	Calories
Subway	Chicken Tortilla Soup (10 oz.), 6-Inch Black Forest Ham Sandwich on 9-Grain Wheat Bread with lettuce, tomatoes, onions, green peppers, cucumbers, and mustard	410
Subway	Fire Roasted Tomato Orzo Soup (10 oz.), 6-Inch Turkey Breast Sandwich on 9-Grain Wheat Bread with lettuce, tomatoes, onions, green peppers, cucumbers, and mustard	420
Subway	Chicken Tortilla Soup, 6-Inch Roast Beef on 9-Grain Wheat Bread with lettuce, tomatoes, onions, green peppers, and cucumbers	410
Taco Bell	Fresco Chicken Burrito Supreme, side of Black Beans	402
Taco Bell	Fresco Steak Burrito Supreme, side of Black Beans	412
Taco Bell	2 Fresco Grilled Steak Tacos, side of Guacamole	355

Healthier Dinner Options

Restaurant	Meal	Calories
Applebee's	Weight Watchers Creamy Parmesan Chicken	470
Applebee's	Chicken Tortilla Soup (Bowl), Weight Watchers Grilled Jalapeno-Lime Shrimp	510
Burger King	BK Veggie Burger (without cheese or mayo), Side Garden Salad with ½ packet Avocado Ranch Dressing, Apple Slices	485
Chili's	Lighter Choice Classic Sirloin (6 oz.) served with Pico de Gallo and Steamed Broccoli, Corn on the Cob (no butter; from the Kid's Menu), side of Pineapple (from the Kid's Menu)	465
Chili's	Lighter Choice Grilled Chicken Salad, side of Pineapple (from the Kid's Menu)	465
Olive Garden	Minestrone Soup, Venetian Apricot Chicken (dinner portion)	500
Olive Garden	Garden Fresh Salad (hold the dressing; request fresh lemon or vinegar to season), Lasagna Primavera with Grilled Chicken (dinner portion)	480

Restaurant	Meal	Calories
PF Chang's	Cup of Egg Drop Soup, Shanghai Shrimp with Garlic Sauce, Half Portion of Brown Rice, Small Asian Tomato Cucumber Salad (from the Sides Menu)	515
PF Chang's	Sichuan Shrimp (no rice), Thai Basil Green Salad with Ginger Lime Vinaigrette	500
PF Chang's	Cup of Wonton Soup, Shrimp with Lobster Sauce (no rice), Thai Basil Green Salad with Ginger Lime Vinaigrette	510
PF Chang's	Shrimp with Lobster Sauce, Half Portion of Brown Rice, Small Asian Tomato Cucumber Salad (from the Sides Menu)	535
PF Chang's	Shanghai Shrimp with Garlic Sauce, Half Portion of Brown Rice, Small Spinach Stir-Fried with Garlic (from the Sides Menu)	515
Red Lobster	Chilled Jumbo Shrimp Cocktail, Red Lobster Tail (no butter), Side of Fresh Broccoli, Garden Salad with Blueberry Balsamic Vinaigrette	510
Red Lobster	Oven Broiled Flounder, Side of Roasted Vegetable Medley, Garden Salad with Blueberry Balsamic Vinaigrette	510
Ruby Tuesday	Grilled Salmon served with Grilled Zucchini and Roasted Spaghetti Squash (from the Fit & Trim Menu)	483
Ruby Tuesday	Hickory Bourbon Salmon served with Grilled Zucchini and Roasted Spaghetti Squash (from the Fit & Trim Menu)	495
Ruby Tuesday	Petite Grilled Sirloin served with Grilled Zucchini and Roasted Spaghetti Squash (from the Fit & Trim Menu), 1 Garlic Cheese Biscuit (from the Brunch Menu)	464
TGIF	6-oz. Sirloin Steak, Side of Broccoli, Tomato Mozzarella Salad	510
Uno Chicago	Tuscan Pesto Minestrone Soup, House Salad with Grilled Chicken and Fat Free Vinaigrette	490

Activate Your Anti-Aging Diet Now!

1 **Check out dining choices online** Eating out on the *7 Years Younger Anti-Aging Breakthrough Diet* is easy. Do your homework by checking out calorie counts online and selecting your dining choices even before you see a menu. Then visualize yourself at the restaurant ordering and eating your healthy choices.

2 **Beware of hidden calories in salads** A salad can be a great meal option, but you have to choose carefully if you want to lose weight. You can never be sure how much oil has gone into a pre-dressed salad— and it's probably a lot more than you think. In addition, watch out for things like cheese, nuts, and avocado; if those ingredients are piled higher than on any salad you had on the *7 Years Younger Anti-Aging Breakthrough Diet* plan, you can push some of the extras to the side to keep your weight loss on track. Salad bars are your best bet, because there you have total control over what goes in and on top of your meal.

3 **Celebrate yourself** Whether you're going out for a special occasion or because you feel like you've earned a night out, focus on enjoying the whole experience, not just the food. The more you savor the restaurant, the company, and the pleasure of being out, the easier it will be to make choices you'll be proud of in the morning.

For more expert diet anti-aging advice, get our free special report Eat to Look & Feel Younger *at 7yearsyounger.com/eattolookyoung.*

Chapter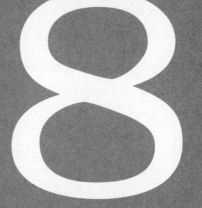

Anti-Aging (& Delicious) Recipes

Pulled Pork on a Bun; a New York Bagel breakfast; Cheesy Chili; Steak & Oven Fries; Asian Chicken Salad; a Sweet Stuffed Waffle with apricot preserves and ricotta. Yum! These are all recipes on the *7 Years Younger Anti-Aging Breakthrough Diet,* a plan that is all about enjoyment.

Our panel of dieters can attest to how delicious these recipes are. They loved the food. Our nutritionists, recipe developers, and recipe testers, under the direction of Good Housekeeping Research Institute Nutrition Director Samantha Cassetty, M.S., R.D., and Food Director Susan Westmoreland spent months in the Test Kitchens working with the team to find the most nutritious and tastiest foods and come up with the ideal menu. We tested the dishes and, if they were too complex, we tossed them aside and started over. We ended up with a menu that includes nearly 100 different ingredients, so there is plenty of variety and lots of opportunity to try new tastes.

Just Loving the Food

The opportunity to communicate with other dieters was an important motivator for our test panelists. Beyond cheering each other on, their biggest discussions focused on how much they were enjoying the recipes. These are just a few examples of what they had to say:

"I made the Steak & Oven Fries for dinner last night," said Porscha Burke. "What an incredible recipe. And the Chicken Parm Stacks are fantastic."

"Last night I made the Healthy-Makeover Meatloaf, and it was amazing," said Robin Greenberg. "My husband loved it."

The reason we're so confident you're going to love these dishes is that they are not "diet" recipes. You'll lunch on terrific sandwiches, savor easy ethnic cuisine at dinner, and eat filling snacks like nuts and pudding. There's even chocolate on the menu. The recipes were created with you in mind—someone who wants food that tastes great, is easy and fast to prepare, appeals to the whole family, and makes you get up from the table with a satisfied stomach and a smile on your face. There's no long list of ingredients or need to spend hours dicing and slicing. Most dishes can be prepared in 30 minutes or less, and all of the dinners were triple-tested in our test kitchens, making them virtually foolproof.

Sitting down nightly at the dinner table is one of the most important bonding rituals a family can participate in. To help enhance the experience, think about some of the strategies we told you about in Chapter 3: Eat more slowly. Put your fork down and appreciate the taste and texture of the food. Notice the nuances—a bit of spice, a hint of sweetness. Record

"I actually love eating lunch, and there have been so many good ones," said Amy Murray, who dropped 16½ pounds and 5¼ inches. "I had the Grilled Mozzarella & Tomato Soup. It was the first time in years that I didn't feel guilty eating grilled cheese."

"My best moments are learning the new recipes and just loving them," said Maggie Patrick, who whittled away 6½ pounds. "At first I was worried that between-meals time would be tough, but I was wrong. The meals are filling," said Mary Marotta, who lost 19 pounds. "I made the Big Fusilli Bowl recipe last night, and it felt like I was cheating."

"My wife, who does most of the cooking, joined me as an unofficial member of our group," said David Sigman. "She has been impressed by the quality of the recipes as well as the quantity of food."

the recipes you like the best in your food diary, as they are the ones you'll want to come back to time and time again.

Most of the 16 breakfasts, 36 lunches, and 24 snack recipes serve one or two; the 64 dinner recipes and mini recipes, four. They are easy to cut in half if you have fewer mouths to feed or increase if you have more.

Don't be concerned that meal prep will make you spend too much time with food and entice you to sneak bites. It's more likely that making your meals will be to your advantage. A University of Minnesota study of 200 dieters found that those who cooked their own meals took in 354 fewer calories per day than those who rarely set foot in the kitchen. Their waists were also more than half an inch smaller, and they had a lower BMI (body mass index)—25.5, versus 26.9. The researchers theorized that when people cooked for themselves and their families, they were more likely to use nutritious foods and limit high-calorie ingredients.

So put on your apron, sharpen your chopping knife, and get cooking!

The Plan

Women: 1,450 calories a day on the main plan
Week 1: 1,200 calories. No snacks

Men *(slightly to moderately active)*:
1,575 calories a day
(Follow the main plan + double the portion of one snack per day)
Week 1: 1,450 calories. Have two snacks per day without doubling portions.

Men *(highly active)*: 1,700 calories a day
(Follow the main plan + double the portions of two snacks per day)
Week 1: 1,575 calories. Have two snacks per day, doubling the portions of one.

Note: Side dishes and desserts serve one; to accommodate additional family members, portions may be increased or substitutes may be served.

BREAKFAST (about 300 calories)

Breakfast Pizza

Split and toast 1 whole-grain English muffin. Top each half with 2 tablespoons part-skim ricotta, 1 thick tomato slice, and black pepper. Drizzle with ½ teaspoon olive oil. On the side: 1 pear.

Each serving about: 292 calories, 10 g protein, 53 g carbohydrate, 6 g total fat (2 g saturated fat), 10 mg cholesterol, 262 mg sodium, 11 mg vitamin C, 163 mg calcium, 9 g fiber, 40 mg omega-3

Breakfast to Go

Have 1 Kind Nuts & Spices bar in Madagascar Vanilla Almond with 1 medium apple.

Each serving about: 305 calories, 7 g protein, 39 g carbohydrate, 16 g total fat (2 g saturated fat), 0 mg cholesterol, 17 mg sodium, 8 mg vitamin C, 11 mg calcium, 9 g fiber, 20 mg omega-3

California Breakfast Bruschetta

Mash ½ Hass avocado with ½ teaspoon lemon juice; spread onto 1 large slice whole-grain toast; top with 1 egg cooked over easy in a skillet coated with cooking spray; sprinkle with ⅛ teaspoon salt.

Each serving about: 302 calories, 12 g protein, 20 g carbohydrate, 21 g total fat (4 g saturated fat), 212 mg cholesterol, 477 mg sodium, 11 mg vitamin C, 66 mg calcium, 9 g fiber, 220 mg omega-3

Easy Oatmeal

Mix 1 packet plain instant oatmeal with ¾ cup fat-free milk and cook as directed. To cooked oatmeal, add ½ banana, sliced; 2 tablespoons chopped walnuts; and 1 teaspoon sugar-free pancake syrup.

Each serving about: 313 calories, 13 g protein, 44 g carbohydrate, 12 g total fat (1 g saturated fat), 4 mg cholesterol, 158 mg sodium, 5 mg vitamin C, 347 mg calcium, 6 g fiber, 1,350 mg omega-3

Grab & Go

Spread 1 tablespoon Philadelphia ⅓ Less Fat Chive & Onion Cream Cheese over both halves of 1 toasted 100% Whole Wheat Thomas' Bagel Thin. Enjoy with a wedge of honeydew melon (⅛ of a large melon) and a 12-ounce nonfat latte.

Each serving about: 302 calories, 20 g protein, 50 g carbohydrate, 5 g total fat (2 g saturated fat), 16 mg cholesterol, 433 mg sodium, 41 mg vitamin C, 460 mg calcium, 6 g fiber, 80 mg omega-3

New York Bagel

Toast one 100% Whole Wheat Thomas' Bagel Thin; spread each half with 1 tablespoon reduced-fat cream cheese. To one half, add 1 ounce lox and 4 tomato slices. Sandwich together and serve. Have with 1 cup honeydew melon.

Each serving about: 285 calories, 15 g protein, 43 g carbohydrate, 9 g total fat (4 g saturated fat), 27 mg cholesterol, 911 mg sodium, 38 mg vitamin C, 79 mg calcium, 7 g fiber, 190 mg omega-3

Peach Melba Yogurt

Stir 1 peach, finely diced (or 1 cup thawed frozen peach slices), and 1/8 teaspoon pure vanilla extract into 1 cup plain fat-free Greek yogurt; top with 1/3 cup fresh or thawed frozen raspberries (mashed or whole) and 3 tablespoons sliced almonds.

Each serving about: 302 calories, 25 g protein, 33 g carbohydrate, 9 g total fat (1 g saturated fat), 0 mg cholesterol, 87 mg sodium, 20 mg vitamin C, 323 mg calcium, 7 g fiber, 50 mg omega-3

Sunrise Soft Taco

Scramble 1 egg and 2 egg whites with 2 tablespoons shredded reduced-fat Monterey Jack cheese; stir in 1/2 cup fresh baby spinach; wrap in an 8-inch (soft taco–size) whole wheat tortilla with 1 tablespoon salsa. Serve with 3/4 cup low-sodium tomato or vegetable juice.

Each serving about: 309 calories, 23 g protein, 34 g carbohydrate, 9 g total fat (3 g saturated fat), 222 mg cholesterol, 627 mg sodium, 58 mg vitamin C, 217 mg calcium, 3 g fiber, 40 mg omega-3

Strawberry Cereal

Combine 1¼ cups Multi-Grain Cheerios cereal with 1¼ cups fat-free milk; top with 5 large strawberries, sliced (about 1/2 cup), and 5 almonds, chopped.

Each serving about: 304 calories, 15 g protein, 52 g carbohydrate, 5 g total fat (1 g saturated fat), 6 mg cholesterol, 388 mg sodium, 55 mg vitamin C, 539 mg calcium, 5 g fiber, 60 mg omega-3

Sweet Stuffed Waffle

Toast two Van's 8 Whole Grains Waffles. On one waffle, spread 1 tablespoon low-sugar apricot preserves and 1/4 cup part-skim ricotta. Top with remaining waffle.

Each serving about: 271 calories, 11 g protein, 38 g carbohydrate, 12 g total fat (4 g saturated fat), 19 mg cholesterol, 308 mg sodium, 0 mg vitamin C, 189 mg calcium, 7 g fiber, 40 mg omega-3

Banana–Peanut Butter Smoothie

Total time 5 minutes • **Makes** 1 serving

    1 small ripe banana, cut in half
    ½ cup low-fat (1%) milk
    1 teaspoon creamy peanut butter
    3 ice cubes

In blender, combine banana, milk, peanut butter, and ice cubes; blend until mixture is smooth and frothy. Makes about 1½ cups.

SIDE FOR ONE Spread 1 slice whole-grain toast with 2 tablespoons part-skim ricotta cheese; top with ½ teaspoon honey and sprinkle with a dash of cinnamon or pumpkin-pie spice.

Nutrition Facts
Each serving about:

Calories	296	Total fat	8 g	Vitamin C	9 mg
		Saturated fat	3 g	Calcium	267 mg
Protein	14 g	Cholesterol	16 mg	Fiber	5 g
Carbohydrate	46 g	Sodium	227 mg	Omega-3	100 mg

Berry Blast Breakfast Shake

Total time 5 minutes • **Makes** 1 serving

    1 container (6 ounces) plain low-fat yogurt
    1 cup frozen berry medley (strawberries, raspberries,
      blackberries, and blueberries)
    ⅓ cup fat-free (skim) milk
    2 tablespoons instant nonfat dry milk powder
    1 tablespoon no-sugar-added strawberry, peach, or apricot jam

In blender, combine yogurt, berries, milk, milk powder, and jam; blend until smooth and frothy. Pour into 1 tall glass.

Nutrition Facts
Each serving about:

Calories	304	Total fat	3 g	Vitamin C	26 mg
		Saturated fat	2 g	Calcium	642 mg
Protein	19 g	Cholesterol	15 mg	Fiber	9 g
Carbohydrate	50 g	Sodium	234 mg	Omega-3	20 mg

5-Minute Multigrain Cereal

Total time 5 minutes · **Makes** 1 serving

- **2 tablespoons quick-cooking barley**
- **2 tablespoons bulgur**
- **2 tablespoons old-fashioned oats**
- **²/₃ cup fat-free milk**
- **2 teaspoons raisins**
- **1 pinch ground cinnamon**
- **1 tablespoon chopped walnuts**
  or pecans

In microwave-safe 1-quart bowl, combine barley, bulgur, oats, and milk. Microwave on High 2 minutes. Stir in raisins and cinnamon; microwave 3 minutes longer. Stir, then top with walnuts.

Nutrition Facts
Each serving about:

Calories	307	Total fat	6 g	Vitamin C	0 mg
Protein	12 g	Saturated fat	1 g	Calcium	228 mg
Carbohydrate	52 g	Cholesterol	3 mg	Fiber	8 g
		Sodium	73 mg	Omega-3	660 mg

Ham & Veggie Hash

Total time 20 minutes · **Makes** 4 servings

6 medium (1½ pounds) red potatoes

1½ pounds green beans

4 ounces thick-sliced ham or ¼ pound cooked ham, in one piece

1 medium red bell pepper

1 medium onion

2 tablespoons vegetable oil

Salt

1 tablespoon chopped fresh parsley

1. Cut potatoes into ½-inch cubes. Trim ends from green beans; cut into 1-inch pieces. In 3-quart saucepan over high heat, heat potatoes, green beans, and enough water to cover to boiling. Reduce heat to low; cover and simmer 2 minutes or until vegetables are almost tender. Drain.

2. Meanwhile, dice ham. In nonstick 12-inch skillet over medium-high heat, cook ham until browned; remove to plate. Chop pepper and onion.

3. In same skillet in hot oil, cook pepper and onion until lightly browned. Add potato-and-green-bean mixture and ½ teaspoon salt and cook, stirring occasionally, until vegetables are tender and browned. Sprinkle with ham and parsley. Adjust seasoning to taste.

Nutrition Facts

Each serving about:

Calories	280	Total fat	8 g	Vitamin C	59 mg
Protein	11 g	Saturated fat	1 g	Calcium	72 mg
Carbohydrate	40 g	Cholesterol	13 mg	Fiber	8 g
		Sodium	624 mg	Omega-3	30 mg

Huevos Rancheros

Total time 25 minutes · **Makes** 4 servings

1 tablespoon vegetable oil

1 medium onion, finely chopped

2 cloves garlic, crushed with press

1 tablespoon chipotle sauce or other hot sauce, plus additional for serving

1 teaspoon ground cumin

1 can (28 ounces) tomatoes in juice, drained and chopped

1 can (15 ounces) black beans, rinsed and drained

¼ cup (loosely packed) fresh cilantro leaves, chopped

Salt

2 teaspoons margarine or butter

4 large eggs

4 (6-inch) corn tortillas, warmed

1. In 4-quart saucepan, heat oil on medium until hot. Add onion and garlic and cook 8 minutes or until beginning to brown. Stir in chipotle sauce and cumin; cook 30 seconds, stirring. Add tomatoes; cover and cook 3 minutes to blend flavors, stirring occasionally. Stir in beans, half of cilantro, and ¼ teaspoon salt; heat through, about 3 minutes, stirring occasionally.

2. Meanwhile, in 12-inch nonstick skillet, melt margarine on medium. Crack eggs, 1 at a time, and drop into skillet. Cover skillet and cook eggs 4 to 5 minutes or until whites are set and yolks thicken.

3. Place tortillas on 4 plates; top each with some tomato mixture and 1 egg. Sprinkle with remaining cilantro.

Nutrition Facts

Each serving about:

Calories	328	Total fat	12 g	Vitamin C	33 mg
		Saturated fat	3 g	Calcium	143 mg
Protein	15 g	Cholesterol	217 mg	Fiber	8 g
Carbohydrate	39 g	Sodium	1,044 mg	Omega-3	50 mg

Smoked-Salmon Scrambled Eggs

Total time 15 minutes · **Makes** 6 servings

10 large eggs

⅓ cup low-fat (1%) milk

¼ cup snipped fresh chives

Pepper

2 teaspoons margarine or butter

5 ounces thinly sliced smoked salmon, cut crosswise into ½-inch strips

1. In large bowl, whisk eggs, milk, 3 tablespoons chives, and ¼ teaspoon freshly ground black pepper until blended.

2. In 12-inch nonstick skillet, melt margarine on medium. Add egg mixture to skillet. As egg mixture begins to set around edge, move it gently toward center with spatula to allow uncooked egg to flow toward side of pan. When eggs are partially cooked, after about 5 minutes, add salmon; cook 1 minute longer or until egg mixture is set but still moist, stirring occasionally. Sprinkle with remaining chives to serve.

SIDE FOR ONE 2 slices whole-grain melba toast and 1 kiwifruit.

Nutrition Facts
Each serving about:

Calories	301	Total fat	12 g	Vitamin C	74 mg
Protein	27 g	Saturated fat	3 g	Calcium	86 mg
Carbohydrate	21 g	Cholesterol	396 mg	Fiber	3 g
		Sodium	236 mg	Omega-3	600 mg

LUNCH (about 400 calories)

Caprese Salad

Toss together 15 grape tomatoes, halved; 1 ounce part-skim mozzarella, cut into chunks; and 3 fresh basil leaves, chopped. Sprinkle with 1 teaspoon each olive oil and balsamic vinegar. On the side: ¼ cup hummus topped with 2 teaspoons pine nuts and served with half of a whole wheat pita, sliced for dipping.

Each serving about: 390 calories, 18 g protein, 39 g carbohydrate, 20 g total fat (5 g saturated fat), 18 mg cholesterol, 597 mg sodium, 33 mg vitamin C, 281 mg calcium, 9 g fiber, 110 mg omega-3

Cheesy Chili

Cook 1 pouch Tabatchnick Vegetarian Chili according to package directions. Sprinkle with 3 tablespoons reduced-fat Cheddar cheese. Serve with 1 ounce (about 16) baked tortilla chips and 2 tablespoons guacamole.

Each serving about: 385 calories, 21 g protein, 56 g carbohydrate, 11 g total fat (2 g saturated fat), 4 mg cholesterol, 839 mg sodium, 8 mg vitamin C, 198 mg calcium, 12 g fiber, 10 mg omega-3

Chinese Rice Bowl

To one container cooked Minute Ready to Serve Brown Rice, add ¼ cup shelled edamame (cooked) and ½ red bell pepper, diced. Toss with ½ teaspoon sesame oil, ½ teaspoon rice vinegar, and 1 teaspoon reduced-sodium soy sauce. Top with ½ teaspoon sesame seeds.

Each serving about: 386 calories, 16 g protein, 56 g carbohydrate, 10 g total fat (1 g saturated fat), 0 mg cholesterol, 410 mg sodium, 95 mg vitamin C, 85 mg calcium, 8 g fiber, 20 mg omega-3

Chipotle Lunch

One serving of Chipotle Mexican Grill salad with lettuce, chicken, black beans, fajita vegetables, and corn salsa; no dressing.

Each serving about: 420 calories, 44 g protein, 45 g carbohydrate, 10 g total fat (2 g saturated fat), 115 mg cholesterol, 1,205 mg sodium, 44 mg vitamin C, 100 mg calcium, 16 g fiber, 0 mg omega-3

Cold Peanut Noodles with Chicken

Toss 1 cup cooked chilled whole wheat linguine with 2 tablespoons orange juice, 1 teaspoon sesame oil, 3 ounces shredded chilled rotisserie-chicken breast meat, 1 cup coleslaw mix, and 15 dry-roasted unsalted peanuts. Sprinkle with 1½ teaspoons reduced-sodium soy sauce and 1 tablespoon fresh cilantro leaves, chopped (optional).

Each serving about: 400 calories, 26 g protein, 44 g carbohydrate, 14 g total fat (2 g saturated fat), 44 mg cholesterol, 921 mg sodium, 32 mg vitamin C, 39 mg calcium, 7 g fiber, 10 mg omega-3

Creole Chicken Frankfurter Meal

Prepare 1 Applegate Farms Organic Chicken Hot Dog according to package directions; serve in a whole wheat frankfurter bun along with 2 tablespoons minced white onion and 1½ teaspoons Creole or spicy mustard. Pair with 1 small microwave-baked sweet potato, sliced, topped with 1 teaspoon butter. Serve with 1 cup watermelon cubes or 1 kiwifruit.

Each serving about: 392 calories, 15 g protein, 61 g carbohydrate, 10 g total fat (4 g saturated fat), 45 mg cholesterol, 776 mg sodium, 75 mg vitamin C, 116 mg calcium, 10 g fiber, 90 mg omega-3

Finger Food

Serve 7 cooked Applegate Farms Chicken Nuggets (180 calories) with hot sauce for dipping. Have with 2 stalks celery served with 2 tablespoons reduced-fat ranch dressing along with 1 ounce (about 15) sweet-potato chips.

Each serving about: 401 calories, 13 g protein, 39 g carbohydrate, 21 g total fat (3 g saturated fat), 41 mg cholesterol, 1,344 mg sodium, 30 mg vitamin C, 98 mg calcium, 3 g fiber, 510 mg omega-3

Greek Feast

Mix ½ cup chickpeas with 5 grape tomatoes, quartered; ½ cucumber, peeled and chopped; 1 teaspoon fresh dill, chopped, or ½ teaspoon dried dill; 2 tablespoons reduced-fat feta; and 2 tablespoons nonfat Greek yogurt. Stuff in a large whole wheat pita.

Each serving about: 376 calories, 21 g protein, 64 g carbohydrate, 6 g total fat (2 g saturated fat), 5 mg cholesterol, 597 mg sodium, 14 mg vitamin C, 149 mg calcium, 13 g fiber, 70 mg omega-3

Grilled Chicken Sandwich

Spread 1½ teaspoons Dijon mustard on a whole wheat hamburger bun and stuff with 3 ounces grilled chicken-breast cutlet (from deli or leftovers), ¾ ounce reduced-fat Cheddar cheese (one slice from a package of presliced cheese), and ½ cup mixed baby greens. Serve with 6 baby carrots and 6 sweet-potato chips.

Each serving about: 405 calories, 37 g protein, 35 g carbohydrate, 13 g total fat (4 g saturated fat), 84 mg cholesterol, 681 mg sodium, 4 mg vitamin C, 277 mg calcium, 7 g fiber, 130 mg omega-3

Grilled Mozzarella & Tomato Soup

Place 1½ ounces part-skim mozzarella cheese and 3 thin tomato slices, and drizzle ½ teaspoon balsamic vinegar, between 2 slices of whole wheat bread. Spritz with olive oil cooking spray, grill in a nonstick skillet over medium-high heat until toasted, and rub the toasted sandwich with half a clove of garlic. Serve with 1 cup Campbell's 100% Natural Harvest Tomato with Basil Soup. Dessert: 2 dried figs.

Each serving about: 398 calories, 18 g protein, 59 g carbohydrate, 9 g total fat (5 g saturated fat), 27 mg cholesterol, 896 mg sodium, 7 mg vitamin C, 439 mg calcium, 8 g fiber, 170 mg omega-3

Ham & Swiss

Spread 1 teaspoon spicy brown mustard on an Arnold Select 100% Whole Wheat Sandwich Thin. Layer with 2 ounces lean lower-sodium ham, ¾ ounce reduced-fat Swiss cheese (one slice from a package of presliced cheese), and 1 romaine lettuce leaf. Dessert: One medium banana, sliced lengthwise, spread with 1 teaspoon natural peanut butter and 1 teaspoon mini chocolate chips. Serve sandwiched together.

Each serving about: 388 calories, 25 g protein, 55 g carbohydrate, 10 g total fat (3 g saturated fat), 40 mg cholesterol, 772 mg sodium, 12 mg vitamin C, 410 mg calcium, 9 g fiber, 40 mg omega-3

Jambalaya

Slice 1 precooked garlic chicken-sausage link and heat; toss with 1 container Minute Ready to Serve Brown Rice; 1 plum tomato, chopped; and ¼ red bell pepper and ¼ green bell pepper, chopped. Season with hot-pepper sauce.

Each serving about: 406 calories, 20 g protein, 49 g carbohydrate, 13 g total fat (3 g saturated fat), 75 mg cholesterol, 850 mg sodium, 73 mg vitamin C, 31 mg calcium, 5 g fiber, 10 mg omega-3

Mediterranean Hummus "Pizza"

Spread ⅓ cup hummus on a fresh or lightly toasted whole wheat pocketless pita or a La Tortilla Factory Smart & Delicious 100% Whole Wheat Flatbread; top with 5 rehydrated sun-dried tomatoes (not oil-packed), thinly sliced; 3 large black olives, thinly sliced; 1 tablespoon fresh basil, thinly sliced; and 2 teaspoons pine nuts. Cut into wedges.

Each serving about: 397 calories, 20 g protein, 53 g carbohydrate, 17 g total fat (2 g saturated fat), 0 mg cholesterol, 826 mg sodium, 3 mg vitamin C, 289 mg calcium, 15 g fiber, 30 mg omega-3

Mediterranean Vegetarian Wrap

On a large soft thin whole-grain flatbread or a (10-inch) whole-grain tortilla, spread ¼ cup hummus; top with 1 ounce reduced-fat feta cheese, 1½ cups packed salad greens, ½ jarred roasted red bell pepper, and 2 thin slices red onion. Sprinkle with ½ teaspoon dried oregano and 1 teaspoon balsamic vinegar, and wrap. Serve with ½ pear sprinkled with cinnamon and topped with 2 walnut halves, crushed.

Each serving about: 410 calories, 17 g protein, 58 g carbohydrate, 16 g total fat (4 g saturated fat), 8 mg cholesterol, 953 mg sodium, 54 mg vitamin C, 139 mg calcium, 12 g fiber, 380 mg omega-3

Mexican Chicken Salad

Atop 2 cups chopped romaine lettuce, arrange ½ cup each canned drained black beans and shredded precooked or rotisserie chicken breast; 5 cherry tomatoes, quartered; ½ small green bell pepper, diced; and ¼ Hass avocado, diced. Dress with 1 teaspoon each canola oil and lime juice.

Each serving about: 392 calories, 32 g protein, 31 g carbohydrate, 16 g total fat (2 g saturated fat), 60 mg cholesterol, 469 mg sodium, 88 mg vitamin C, 103 mg calcium, 14 g fiber, 640 mg omega-3

Mexican Meal in Minutes

Heat 1 Healthy Choice Chicken Tortilla microwavable soup bowl. Serve with one 6-inch soft corn tortilla wrapped around 2 tablespoons shredded reduced-fat Monterey Jack cheese and 1½ tablespoons bean dip, at room temperature or warmed in the microwave.

Each serving about: 420 calories, 24 g protein, 64 g carbohydrate, 7 g total fat (3 g saturated fat), 38 mg cholesterol, 1,118 mg sodium, 0 mg vitamin C, 240 mg calcium, 12 g fiber, 0 mg omega-3

Microwavable Pasta Meal

1 Healthy Choice Italian Sausage Pasta Bake (270 calories); serve with 2 cups fresh baby spinach tossed with ¼ cup no-salt-added chickpeas, 1 tablespoon Parmesan cheese, and 1 tablespoon reduced-fat balsamic vinaigrette.

Each serving about: 387 calories, 23 g protein, 60 g carbohydrate, 9 g total fat (3 g saturated fat), 19 mg cholesterol, 912 mg sodium, 10 mg vitamin C, 266 mg calcium, 11 g fiber, 10 mg omega-3

No-Cook Bean Burrito

Fill an 8-inch whole wheat tortilla with ½ cup canned refried beans (about 100 calories per ½ cup), ¼ avocado, 2 tablespoons salsa, and ½ slice reduced-fat sharp Cheddar cheese, torn into pieces; roll. Warm in the microwave for 20 to 30 seconds (optional). Serve with 2 cups mixed salad greens and 8 grape tomatoes lightly tossed with 2 teaspoons reduced-fat red-wine vinaigrette.

Each serving about: 434 calories, 18 g protein, 60 g carbohydrate, 15 g total fat (3 g saturated fat), 8 mg cholesterol, 605 mg sodium, 26 mg vitamin C, 196 mg calcium, 17 g fiber, 80 mg omega-3

Peanut Butter & Apple Sandwich

Spread 2 slices whole wheat bread with a total of 1 tablespoon unsalted no-sugar-added natural peanut butter or almond butter. Layer with slices from half of a small apple (save other half for dessert). Serve with 1 cup crudités (e.g., broccoli, cauliflower, or red bell pepper pieces). Dessert: Use remaining apple slices as a side with dip made from ½ cup Greek yogurt mixed with sugar-free maple syrup to taste and a drop of vanilla.

Each serving about: 380 calories, 21 g protein, 52 g carbohydrate, 10 g total fat (1 g saturated fat), 0 mg cholesterol, 369 mg sodium, 7 mg vitamin C, 202 mg calcium, 8 g fiber, 20 mg omega-3

Protein Plate

1 hard-boiled egg served with ¼ cup hummus, 5 grape tomatoes, 15 sugar snap peas, and 3 reduced-fat Triscuits. Have with one small apple, cut into slices and served with 1 stick part-skim mozzarella string cheese.

Each serving about: 397 calories, 21 g protein, 47 g carbohydrate, 17 g total fat (5 g saturated fat), 222 mg cholesterol, 505 mg sodium, 48 mg vitamin C, 88 mg calcium, 11 g fiber, 60 mg omega-3

Roast Beef Chef's Salad

On 3 cups baby spinach leaves, arrange 1 hard-cooked egg, chopped; 3 ounces lean roast beef, cubed; 5 mushrooms, thinly sliced; 3 red onion slices; and 3 tablespoons crumbled reduced-fat feta or shredded Swiss cheese. Dress with 1½ tablespoons reduced-fat balsamic vinaigrette, and season with ¼ teaspoon pepper. Serve with 12 SunChips.

Each serving about: 408 calories, 40 g protein, 30 g carbohydrate, 16 g total fat (6 g saturated fat), 294 mg cholesterol, 843 mg sodium, 15 mg vitamin C, 175 mg calcium, 5 g fiber, 60 mg omega-3

Roast Beef Pockets

Cut a large whole wheat pita in half. Spread each half with 1 teaspoon horseradish mustard and then layer 2 ounces lean roast beef and 1 slice reduced-fat Cheddar cheese between the two halves. Serve with (or stuff the pockets with) 2 cups baby arugula tossed with ¼ cup diced roasted red bell pepper, 2 teaspoons red wine vinegar, and ½ teaspoon extra virgin olive oil.

Each serving about: 385 calories, 29 g protein, 43 g carbohydrate, 12 g total fat (4 g saturated fat), 55 mg cholesterol, 681 mg sodium, 138 mg vitamin C, 361 mg calcium, 6 g fiber, 90 mg omega-3

Sandwich & Slaw

Spread 2 teaspoons light mayonnaise on a whole wheat hamburger bun; layer on 2 ounces thinly sliced low-sodium smoked turkey or ham and 1/3 cup coleslaw. Enjoy with 1 Mini Babybel Light cheese and 10 grapes.

Each serving about: 373 calories, 21 g protein, 42 g carbohydrate, 14 g total fat (3 g saturated fat), 49 mg cholesterol, 925 mg sodium, 22 mg vitamin C, 303 mg calcium, 4 g fiber, 470 mg omega-3

Shrimp Caesar Salad

Toss together 3 cups chopped romaine lettuce with 8 large precooked, chilled shrimp, 5 grape tomatoes, and 2 tablespoons reduced-fat Caesar dressing; sprinkle with 1 tablespoon unsalted pine nuts, 2 tablespoons grated Parmesan cheese, and freshly ground black pepper. Enjoy with 1 (1½-ounce) whole-grain roll and 1 small peach or 2 kiwifruits.

Each serving about: 415 calories, 22 g protein, 46 g carbohydrate, 18 g total fat (4 g saturated fat), 100 mg cholesterol, 894 mg sodium, 47 mg vitamin C, 291 mg calcium, 8 g fiber, 220 mg omega-3

Subway Sandwich & Soup

Have 8 ounces Fire Roasted Tomato Orzo Soup (100 calories) plus one 6-Inch Turkey Breast sandwich on 9-Grain Wheat bread with lettuce, tomatoes, onions, green peppers, cucumbers, and brown mustard (280 calories).

Each serving about: 380 calories, 23 g protein, 65 g carbohydrate, 5 g total fat (1 g saturated fat), 21 mg cholesterol, 1,140 mg sodium, 14 mg vitamin C, 380 mg calcium, 7 g fiber, 0 mg omega-3

Sushi to Go

Have 1 (6-piece) California maki sushi roll (made with brown rice, if available), 1/4 cup dry-roasted edamame with salt, and 1 small mandarin orange.

Each serving about: 393 calories, 24 g protein, 78 g carbohydrate, 7 g total fat (1 g saturated fat), 4 mg cholesterol, 577 mg sodium, 31 mg vitamin C, 80 mg calcium, 14 g fiber, 0 mg omega-3

Veggie Burger

Have a black bean veggie burger, such as MorningStar Farms Spicy Black Bean Veggie Burger, on a whole-grain bun with 3 slices tomato, 1 slice red onion, 2 leaves green leaf lettuce, and 2 tablespoons Wholly Guacamole All Natural Classic Guacamole. Enjoy with a fresh plum or clementine.

Each serving about: 401 calories, 21 g protein, 58 g carbohydrate, 12 g total fat (2 g saturated fat), 2 mg cholesterol, 791 mg sodium, 15 mg vitamin C, 82 mg calcium, 13 g fiber, 0 mg omega-3

Asian Chicken Salad

Active time 20 minutes · **Total time** 30 minutes · **Makes** 5 servings

3 limes

4 medium boneless, skinless chicken-breast halves (1½ pounds)

1 bag (16 ounces) frozen shelled edamame

⅓ cup reduced-sodium soy sauce

¼ cup loosely packed fresh cilantro leaves, chopped

1 tablespoon peeled fresh ginger, grated

2 teaspoons sesame oil

1 pound napa (Chinese) cabbage (½ small head), sliced

1 bunch or 1 bag (6 ounces) radishes, trimmed and thinly sliced

1. Cut 2 limes into thin slices. From remaining lime, squeeze 2 tablespoons juice; set aside.

2. In covered 12-inch skillet, heat half of lime slices and 1 inch water to boiling on high. Add chicken; cover, reduce heat to medium-low, and cook 13 to 14 minutes or until chicken is cooked through (165°F). With slotted spoon or tongs, remove chicken from skillet and place in large bowl of ice water; chill 5 minutes. Drain chicken well; with hands, shred chicken into bite-size pieces.

3. Meanwhile, cook edamame as label directs; drain. Rinse with cold running water to stop cooking, and drain again. In large bowl, whisk together soy sauce, cilantro, ginger, sesame oil, and reserved lime juice. Add cabbage, edamame, radishes, and shredded chicken to bowl; toss to combine.

4. To serve, transfer to deep bowls and garnish with remaining lime slices.

SIDE FOR ONE 12 Planters Smoked Almonds or 24 Planters Sea Salt and Black Pepper Pistachios.

Nutrition Facts
Each serving about:

Calories	414	Total fat	16 g	Vitamin C	50 mg
Protein	43 g	Saturated fat	2 g	Calcium	167 mg
Carbohydrate	23 g	Cholesterol	75 mg	Fiber	9 g
		Sodium	672 mg	Omega-3	60 mg

Chicken Caesar Pitas

Total time 20 minutes · **Makes** 4 servings

2 **tablespoons fresh lemon juice**

1 **tablespoon red wine vinegar**

1 **teaspoon Dijon mustard**

Salt and pepper

1 **teaspoon anchovy paste (optional)**

2½ **tablespoons olive oil**

1 **clove garlic, cut in half**

4 **whole wheat pitas, each cut in half**

1 **romaine lettuce heart, chopped**

¼ **cup fresh basil leaves, sliced**

¼ **cup shredded Parmesan cheese**

1 **cup grape tomatoes, each cut in half**

12 **ounces shredded rotisserie-chicken breast meat**

1. In large bowl, with wire whisk, stir lemon juice, vinegar, mustard, ⅛ teaspoon each salt and freshly ground black pepper, and anchovy paste, if using, until well mixed. While whisking, add oil in slow, steady stream until incorporated.

2. Rub cut sides of garlic all over insides of pitas; discard garlic. Microwave pitas on High 15 seconds.

3. In bowl with dressing, combine lettuce, basil, Parmesan, tomatoes, and chicken, tossing to coat. Divide mixture among pitas.

Nutrition Facts
Each serving about:

Calories	384	Total fat	14 g	Vitamin C	10 mg
		Saturated fat	3 g	Calcium	91 mg
Protein	29 g	Cholesterol	56 mg	Fiber	5 g
Carbohydrate	40 g	Sodium	942 mg	Omega-3	70 mg

Easy Cobb Salad

Total time 25 minutes · **Makes** 6 servings

- **6 slices fully cooked, ready-to-serve bacon**
- **2 bags (5 ounces each) mixed baby greens**
- **1 pint red or yellow cherry or grape tomatoes, each cut in half**
- **2 cups fresh corn kernels (1 ear yields ½ cup)**
- **2 cups (½-inch cubes) skinless cooked chicken meat**
- **½ English (hothouse) cucumber, unpeeled, cut into ¼-inch dice**
- **3 ounces blue cheese, crumbled**
- **⅓ cup reduced-fat balsamic vinaigrette**

1. Heat bacon in microwave oven as label directs; cool slightly, then coarsely chop.

2. Line large, deep platter with baby greens. Arrange cherry tomatoes, corn, chicken, cucumber, blue cheese, and bacon in striped pattern over greens. Serve with vinaigrette.

SIDE FOR ONE 1 (1-ounce) whole-grain soft breadstick or small roll.

DESSERT FOR ONE 1 large bunch red or green seedless grapes (20 grapes).

Nutrition Facts

Each serving about:

Calories	399	Total fat	12 g	Vitamin C	38 mg
		Saturated fat	5 g	Calcium	177 mg
Protein	25 g	Cholesterol	54 mg	Fiber	6 g
Carbohydrate	53 g	Sodium	709 mg	Omega-3	140 mg

Garden Turkey Sandwich with Lemon Mayo

Total time 8 minutes · **Makes** 1 serving

- 1 **teaspoon grated lemon peel**
- 1 **tablespoon light mayonnaise**
- 2 **slices whole-grain bread**

Pepper

- 1 **cup loosely packed baby spinach leaves**
- 3 **ounces smoked turkey breast, sliced**
- 1 **plum tomato, sliced**

1. Stir grated lemon peel into mayonnaise; spread on both bread slices. Sprinkle with ⅛ teaspoon freshly ground black pepper.

2. On 1 bread slice, alternately layer spinach leaves, turkey, and tomato, starting and ending with spinach. Top with second bread slice.

SIDE FOR ONE 10 SunChips.

Nutrition Facts
Each serving about:

Calories	388	Total fat	13 g	Vitamin C	14 mg
Protein	25 g	Saturated fat	3 g	Calcium	82 mg
Carbohydrate	46 g	Cholesterol	44 mg	Fiber	7 g
		Sodium	1,195 mg	Omega-3	380 mg

Open-Face Jarlsberg Sandwiches with Greens

Total time 20 minutes · **Makes** 6 servings

- **2 teaspoons olive oil**
- **1 clove garlic, thinly sliced**
- **1 bag (5 to 6 ounces) baby spinach**

Salt and pepper

- **6 slices (each ½ inch thick) artisanal whole-grain bread (from center of round loaf)**
- **2 tablespoons Dijon mustard**
- **3 (3-ounce) plum tomatoes, sliced**
- **6 ounces Jarlsberg cheese, shredded**

1. Preheat broiler. In 12-inch nonstick skillet, heat oil on medium 1 minute. Add garlic and cook 3 to 4 minutes or until garlic is golden, stirring occasionally. Stir in spinach and cook 1 to 2 minutes or until spinach wilts. Stir in ⅛ teaspoon each salt and freshly ground black pepper. Remove skillet from heat.

2. Meanwhile, place bread on cookie sheet and toast in broiler 2 minutes or until beginning to brown.

3. Turn toasted bread over and spread mustard on top of bread slices; top with spinach, tomatoes, and cheese. Broil sandwiches 2 to 3 minutes or until cheese melts and begins to brown.

SIDE FOR ONE 1 ounce Food Should Taste Good Multigrain Chips or 1 (1.3-ounce) bag Glenny's Multigrain Soy Crisps.

Nutrition Facts

Each serving about:

Calories	393	Total fat	12 g	Vitamin C	8 mg
Protein	17 g	Saturated fat	6 g	Calcium	343 mg
Carbohydrate	42 g	Cholesterol	25 mg	Fiber	8 g
		Sodium	533 mg	Omega-3	80 mg

Southwest Chicken Wraps

Total time 18 minutes · **Makes** 4 servings

2 **teaspoons olive oil**

1 **pound ground chicken-breast or turkey-breast meat**

1 **medium red bell pepper, chopped**

1 **teaspoon chili powder**

1 **teaspoon ground cumin**

Salt

1 **cup mild salsa**

1 **can (15 ounces) pinto beans, rinsed and drained**

12 **Boston lettuce leaves**

⅓ **cup plain nonfat Greek yogurt**

1. In 12-inch nonstick skillet, heat olive oil on medium 1 minute. Add chicken, red pepper, chili powder, ground cumin, and ⅛ teaspoon salt. Cook, stirring occasionally, until chicken loses its pink color throughout, about 8 minutes. Stir in salsa and beans; cook 5 minutes to blend flavors and heat through. Adjust seasoning.

2. Arrange 3 lettuce leaves on each plate. Divide chicken mixture evenly among lettuce-leaf cups. Top each lettuce cup with a dollop of yogurt. Fold leaves over mixture and eat wraps out of hand.

SIDE FOR ONE 5 Food Should Taste Good Blue Corn Tortilla Chips with 1 tablespoon Wholly Guacamole All Natural Classic Guacamole.

Nutrition Facts
Each serving about:

Calories	401	Total fat	15 g	Vitamin C	47 mg
Protein	29 g	Saturated fat	4 g	Calcium	112 mg
Carbohydrate	31 g	Cholesterol	98 mg	Fiber	9 g
		Sodium	259 mg	Omega-3	170 mg

Spicy Black Bean Soup

Total time 40 minutes · **Makes** 6 (⅔-cup) servings

1 tablespoon vegetable oil

1 medium onion, chopped

2 cloves garlic, finely chopped

2 teaspoons chili powder

1 teaspoon ground cumin

¼ teaspoon crushed red pepper

2 cans (15 ounces each) black beans, rinsed and drained

2 cups water

1 can (14½ ounces) chicken broth

1 Hass avocado, pitted, peeled, and diced

¼ cup coarsely chopped fresh cilantro

Lime wedges

1. In 3-quart saucepan, heat oil over medium heat. Add onion and cook, stirring occasionally, until tender, 5 to 8 minutes. Stir in garlic, chili powder, cumin, and crushed red pepper; cook 30 seconds. Stir in beans, water, and broth; heat to boiling over high heat. Reduce heat and simmer 15 minutes.

2. Spoon one-third of mixture into blender; cover, with center part of cover removed to let steam escape, and puree until smooth. Pour puree into bowl. Repeat with remaining mixture. Sprinkle with avocado and cilantro and serve with lime wedges. Freeze leftovers.

OPEN-FACE SANDWICH FOR ONE Top 1 slice whole wheat bread with 1 ounce low-sodium smoked turkey breast; one ¾-ounce slice part-skim mozzarella cheese; ½ cup baby arugula; ¼ avocado, sliced; and a squirt of lemon.

Nutrition Facts

Each serving about:

Calories	398	Total fat	16 g	Vitamin C 39 mg
Protein	24 g	Saturated fat 4 g		Calcium 313 mg
Carbohydrate	40 g	Cholesterol	26 mg	Fiber 14 g
		Sodium	925 mg	Omega-3 120 mg

Spinach & Nectarine Salad

Total time 13 minutes · **Makes** 2 servings

- **2 tablespoons 100%-fruit orange marmalade**
- **1 large shallot, thinly sliced**
- **2 tablespoons white balsamic vinegar**
- **1 tablespoon olive oil**
- **Salt and pepper**
- **¼ cup slivered almonds**
- **1 package (7 ounces) baby spinach**
- **2 ripe nectarines, pitted and cut into wedges**
  (use pears or peaches if you don't have nectarines)

1. In microwave-safe small bowl or 1-cup liquid measuring cup, combine marmalade and shallot. Cover with vented plastic wrap and cook in microwave on High 1 minute. Stir in vinegar, oil, ¼ teaspoon salt, and ¼ teaspoon freshly ground black pepper.

2. In small skillet, cook almonds on medium 5 minutes, stirring until toasted. Set aside to cool, about 2 minutes.

3. To serve, toss spinach, nectarines, and marmalade mixture until combined. Place on 2 dinner plates; scatter almonds on top.

SIDE FOR ONE ½ cup low-fat (1%), low-sodium cottage cheese with pinch of freshly ground black pepper.

Nutrition Facts
Each serving about:

Calories	381	Total fat	15 g	Vitamin C	22 mg
Protein	21 g	Saturated fat	2 g	Calcium	190 mg
Carbohydrate	45 g	Cholesterol	5 mg	Fiber	9 g
		Sodium	467 mg	Omega-3	10 mg

Tuna & Cannellini Bean Salad

Total time 12 minutes · **Makes** 6 servings

1 large lemon

2 cans (15 ounces each) white kidney (cannellini)
  beans, rinsed and drained

1 jar (4 ounces) sliced pimientos, drained

¼ cup loosely packed fresh parsley leaves, chopped

3 tablespoons olive oil

Salt and pepper

1 can (12 ounces) light tuna packed in water, drained and flaked

1 bag (5 to 6 ounces) baby spinach or arugula

1. From lemon, finely grate 1 teaspoon peel and squeeze 3 tablespoons juice.

2. In serving bowl, combine lemon peel and juice, beans, pimientos, parsley, oil, ½ teaspoon salt, and ⅛ teaspoon freshly ground black pepper. Gently stir in tuna; serve with baby spinach.

SIDE FOR ONE 10 Multigrain Wheat Thins and ¾ cup mixed fresh or frozen thawed berries.

Nutrition Facts

Each serving about:

Calories	383	Total fat	12 g	Vitamin C 30 mg
Protein	24 g	Saturated fat	1 g	Calcium 100 mg
Carbohydrate	49 g	Cholesterol	17 mg	Fiber 12 g
		Sodium	420 mg	Omega-3 150 mg

DINNER (about 500 calories)

Big Fusilli Bowl

Total time 30 minutes · **Makes** 4 servings

12 ounces whole-grain fusilli or rotini pasta

1 bag (12 ounces) fresh broccoli florets

1 pint grape tomatoes

2 large garlic cloves, peeled and smashed with side of chef's knife

1½ tablespoons olive oil

Salt and pepper

¼ cup grated Pecorino Romano cheese

½ cup (2 ounces) diced part-skim mozzarella cheese

2 tablespoons thinly sliced fresh basil

1½ tablespoons pine nuts, toasted

1. Preheat oven to 450°F. Heat large covered saucepot of salted water to boiling on high. Add pasta and cook as label directs, adding broccoli when 3 minutes of cooking time remain.

2. Meanwhile, in bowl, toss tomatoes with garlic, oil, and ¼ teaspoon salt. Spread tomato mixture in 15½" by 10½" jelly-roll pan and roast 15 minutes or until tomatoes wrinkle and begin to burst, stirring halfway through cooking time.

3. Reserve ½ cup pasta cooking water; drain pasta and broccoli. Add reserved pasta cooking water to jelly-roll pan, stirring to scrape up any browned bits. Return pasta and broccoli to saucepot; stir in tomato mixture, Romano, ½ teaspoon salt, and ¼ teaspoon freshly ground black pepper. Sprinkle with mozzarella, basil, and pine nuts.

Nutrition Facts

Each serving about:					
Calories	480	Total fat	14 g	Vitamin C	90 mg
Protein	23 g	Saturated fat	4 g	Calcium	293 mg
Carbohydrate	73 g	Cholesterol	18 mg	Fiber	11 g
		Sodium	808 mg	Omega-3	200 mg

Garden-Vegetable Omelet

Active time 30 minutes · **Total time** 45 minutes · **Makes** 4 servings

8 ounces red potatoes,
cut into ½-inch pieces

1 onion, finely chopped

1 red bell pepper, cut into ½-inch pieces

1 green bell pepper, cut into ½-inch pieces

1 small zucchini (8 ounces),
cut into ½-inch pieces

Salt and pepper

¼ cup water

4 tablespoons chopped fresh basil leaves

6 large egg whites

2 large eggs

½ cup (2 ounces) crumbled feta cheese

1. In small saucepan, heat potatoes and enough water to cover to boiling over high heat. Reduce heat to low; cover and simmer until tender, about 10 minutes. Drain.

2. Spray nonstick 12-inch skillet with nonstick cooking spray. Add onion and cook over medium heat 5 minutes. Add red and green pepper, zucchini, ½ teaspoon salt, and ¼ teaspoon freshly ground black pepper and cook, stirring frequently, until vegetables are tender-crisp. Stir in water and heat to boiling. Reduce to low; cover and simmer 10 minutes or until vegetables are tender. Remove skillet from heat; stir in potatoes and 1 tablespoon basil.

3. Preheat oven to 375°F. In medium bowl, with wire whisk or fork, mix egg whites, eggs, ¼ cup feta, and remaining 3 tablespoons basil.

4. Spray oven-safe 10-inch skillet with nonstick cooking spray. Pour egg mixture into pan and cook over medium-high heat until it begins to set, 1 to 2 minutes. Remove skillet from heat. With slotted spoon, spread vegetable mixture over egg mixture in skillet; sprinkle with remaining ¼ cup feta. Bake until omelet sets, about 10 minutes. If you like, broil 1 to 2 minutes to brown top of omelet.

SIDE FOR ONE 3 cups baby arugula tossed with 3 tablespoons raisins and 2 tablespoons each toasted chopped walnuts and crumbled feta cheese, 1½ teaspoons vegetable oil, and fresh lemon juice to taste.

Nutrition Facts

Each serving about:

Calories	491	Total fat	26 g	Vitamin C	115 mg
Protein	20 g	Saturated fat	7 g	Calcium	319 mg
Carbohydrate	50 g	Cholesterol	118 mg	Fiber	7 g
		Sodium	762 mg	Omega-3	2,230 mg

Spaghetti with Pesto Verde

Total time 30 minutes · **Makes** 4 servings

  6 **ounces baby spinach**
10 **ounces frozen broccoli florets**
  1 **clove garlic, peeled**
  2 **medium zucchini, trimmed**
  2 **medium tomatoes, cored**
  8 **ounces whole-grain spaghetti**
  1 **cup fresh basil leaves**
  2 **tablespoons fresh lemon juice**
  2 **tablespoons pine nuts**
Salt and pepper
¼ **cup extra virgin olive oil**
  1 **ounce Parmesan cheese, freshly grated**

1. Heat large covered saucepot of salted water to boiling on high.

2. In microwave-safe bowl, combine spinach, broccoli, garlic, and 1 cup water. Cover with vented plastic wrap and microwave on High 3 to 5 minutes or until broccoli is thawed and spinach is tender. Drain; let cool completely.

3. Meanwhile, with vegetable peeler, peel zucchini into wide ribbons. Chop tomatoes.

4. Cook spaghetti as label directs.

5. Place cooled broccoli mixture, basil, lemon juice, pine nuts, and ¼ teaspoon each salt and freshly ground black pepper in food processor; pulse until smooth. With processor running, drizzle in oil. Add Parmesan; pulse until well combined.

6. Drain spaghetti well and return to pot; add pesto, zucchini, tomatoes, and ¼ teaspoon salt; toss well. Serve immediately.

DESSERT FOR ONE ½ cup fresh cherries or raspberries.

Nutrition Facts
Each serving about:

Calories	491	Total fat	20 g	Vitamin C	52 mg
Protein	15 g	Saturated fat	4 g	Calcium	187 mg
Carbohydrate	67 g	Cholesterol	6 mg	Fiber	14 g
		Sodium	201 mg	Omega-3	200 mg

Two-Cheese Pita Pizzas with Broccoli & Tomato

Total time 35 minutes · **Makes** 4 servings

1 tablespoon olive oil

1 medium red onion, sliced

2 cloves garlic, crushed with press

¼ teaspoon crushed red pepper

8 ounces broccoli florets, cut into 1½-inch pieces

Salt

1 can (15 ounces) garbanzo beans, rinsed and drained

1 cup part-skim ricotta cheese

4 (6-inch) whole wheat pitas, each split horizontally in half

⅓ cup grated Parmesan cheese

2 medium plum tomatoes, cut into ½-inch chunks

1. Preheat oven to 450°F. In nonstick 12-inch skillet, heat oil over medium-high heat until hot. Add onion and cook 7 to 10 minutes or until golden, stirring occasionally. Add garlic and crushed red pepper and cook 30 seconds, stirring. Add broccoli florets, ¼ teaspoon salt, and ¼ cup water; heat to boiling. Reduce heat to medium and cook, covered, 5 minutes or until broccoli is tender-crisp.

2. Meanwhile, in small bowl, with potato masher or fork, mash beans with ricotta and ¼ teaspoon salt until almost smooth.

3. Arrange pita halves on 2 large cookie sheets. Bake 3 minutes or until lightly toasted. Spread bean mixture on toasted pitas. Top with broccoli mixture and sprinkle with Parmesan. Bake 7 to 10 minutes longer or until heated through. Sprinkle with tomatoes to serve.

DESSERT FOR ONE ½ cup frozen green or red seedless grapes.

Nutrition Facts

Each serving about:

Calories	494	Total fat	14 g	Vitamin C	68 mg
		Saturated fat	5 g	Calcium	332 mg
Protein	24 g	Cholesterol	25 mg	Fiber	12 g
Carbohydrate	75 g	Sodium	1,019 mg	Omega-3	190 mg

Ziti with Peas, Grape Tomatoes & Ricotta

Total time 35 minutes · **Makes** 6 servings

2 pounds fresh peas in the pod or 2 cups frozen peas, thawed
14 ounces whole-grain ziti or penne rigate pasta
1 cup part-skim ricotta cheese
¼ cup loosely packed fresh parsley leaves, chopped
¼ cup Romano cheese, freshly grated
2 teaspoons fresh lemon peel (from 1 lemon), grated
Salt and pepper
2 teaspoons olive oil
1 pint grape tomatoes

1. Heat large covered saucepot of salted water to boiling over high heat.

2. Meanwhile, if using fresh peas, shell by running thumb along length of each pod's seam to open pod and release peas.

3. Add pasta to boiling water and cook as label directs. Add fresh peas to saucepot when pasta has 2 minutes cooking time remaining. (Add frozen peas when pasta has 1 minute left to cook.)

4. While pasta is cooking, in medium bowl, combine ricotta, parsley, Romano, lemon peel, ½ teaspoon salt, and ¼ teaspoon freshly ground black pepper; set aside. In 12-inch skillet, heat oil over medium-high heat. Add tomatoes and cook 6 to 8 minutes or until tomatoes burst and are heated through, shaking pan frequently. Remove skillet from heat.

5. Remove ½ cup pasta cooking water; set aside. Drain pasta and peas.

6. To skillet with tomatoes, add pasta with peas and reserved pasta cooking water; stir to combine. Spoon into 6 bowls and dollop with ricotta mixture.

DESSERT FOR ONE One ½-cup scoop Edy's Slow Churned No Sugar Added Ice Cream, Neapolitan flavor (90 calories), with 3 walnut halves crumbled on top.

Nutrition Facts

Each serving about:

Calories	503	Total fat	15 g	Vitamin C	30 mg
Protein	23 g	Saturated fat	6 g	Calcium	333 mg
Carbohydrate	75 g	Cholesterol	29 mg	Fiber	11 g
		Sodium	491 mg	Omega-3	620 mg

Basil-Orange Chicken with Couscous

Active time 20 minutes · **Total time** 30 minutes · **Makes** 4 servings

2 large navel oranges

3 lemons

½ cup packed chopped fresh
  basil leaves

2 tablespoons olive oil

Salt and pepper

4 skinless, boneless chicken-breast
  halves (1½ pounds)

½ teaspoon sugar (optional)

1 cup whole wheat couscous

1 package (8 ounces) stringless sugar snap peas

¼ cup natural almond slices, toasted

1. From 1 orange, grate 1½ teaspoons peel and squeeze 4 tablespoons juice. From 2 lemons, grate 1½ teaspoons peel and squeeze ⅓ cup juice. Cut remaining orange and lemon into slices and set aside.

2. In medium bowl, combine 1 teaspoon of each peel and 1 tablespoon orange juice with half of basil, 1 tablespoon olive oil, and ¼ teaspoon each salt and frashly ground black pepper.

3. Place chicken between two sheets of plastic wrap and, with flat side of meat mallet, pound to an even ½-inch thickness. Add chicken to citrus mixture, turning to coat; set aside.

4. In small pitcher or bowl, combine sugar (if using) and remaining ⅛ teaspoon pepper, citrus peels, citrus juices, basil, and oil; set aside. (Can be made to this point up to 8 hours ahead: Cover chicken and citrus sauce and refrigerate.)

5. Preheat large ridged grill pan or prepare outdoor grill for direct grilling on medium-high. Meanwhile, prepare couscous as label directs. In 4-quart saucepan filled with ½ inch water, place a vegetable steamer. Heat to boiling on high.

6. Add chicken to hot grill pan or place on hot grill grate; cook 4 minutes. Turn chicken over and cook 3 to 4 minutes longer or until 165°F and no longer pink in center. Grill reserved citrus slices as well.

7. After turning chicken, add snap peas to steamer; cook 2 to 3 minutes or until tender-crisp. Fluff couscous and spoon onto platter; top with chicken and snap peas. Drizzle with sauce. Garnish with almonds and citrus slices.

Nutrition Facts

Each serving about:

Calories	509	Total fat	14 g	Vitamin C	55 mg
Protein	45 g	Saturated fat	2 g	Calcium	128 mg
Carbohydrate	52 g	Cholesterol	94 mg	Fiber	10 g
		Sodium	235 mg	Omega-3	150 mg

Chicken with Berry Sauce

Total time 25 minutes · **Makes** 4 servings

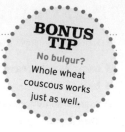

BONUS TIP

No bulgur? Whole wheat couscous works just as well.

  1 teaspoon ground cumin
 ½ teaspoon ground allspice
Salt and pepper
  1 cup bulgur
1¼ pounds chicken-breast cutlets
  1 tablespoon olive oil
 ⅓ cup salted pistachios, roasted
  1 pint blackberries
1½ cups frozen peas, thawed

1. In small bowl, stir together cumin, allspice, and ¼ teaspoon freshly ground black pepper. In large microwave-safe bowl, combine bulgur, 1½ cups water, ½ teaspoon spice mixture, and ⅛ teaspoon salt. Cover with vented plastic wrap and microwave on High 12 minutes or until bulgur is tender.

2. Meanwhile, sprinkle 1 teaspoon spice mixture and ⅛ teaspoon salt all over chicken. In 12-inch nonstick skillet, heat oil on medium 1 minute. Add chicken to pan; cook 8 to 10 minutes or until 165°F and juices run clear, turning over once.

3. While chicken cooks, shell and chop pistachios. Transfer chicken to plate.

4. To same skillet, add blackberries, ¼ cup water, remaining spice mixture, and ⅛ teaspoon salt. With potato masher, gently crush blackberries to release some juice. Cook 3 minutes or until slightly reduced, scraping up browned bits.

5. Fold peas and pistachios into cooked bulgur. Serve with chicken and blackberry sauce.

DESSERT FOR ONE One 4-ounce container Kozy Shack No Sugar Added Chocolate Pudding or other sugar-free pudding (70 calories).

Nutrition Facts
Each serving about:

Calories	483	Total fat	14 g	
		Saturated fat	3 g	
Protein	39 g	Cholesterol	78 mg	
Carbohydrate	55 g	Sodium	328 mg	
Vitamin C	17 mg			
Calcium	93 mg			
Fiber	14 g			
Omega-3	160 mg			

Chicken Lo Mein Primavera

Total time 30 minutes · **Makes** 4 servings

1 package (14 ounces) extra-firm tofu, drained

1 package (9 ounces) fresh whole-grain linguine

2 tablespoons vegetable oil

2 stalks celery, thinly sliced

1 large red bell pepper, thinly sliced

3 cloves garlic, crushed with press

1 large zucchini, cut into ¼-inch-thick half-moons

2 large carrots, shredded

¼ cup reduced-sodium soy sauce

8 ounces precooked chicken-breast strips or pieces

½ teaspoon Asian sesame oil

Fresh cilantro leaves, for garnish

1. Cut tofu block in half lengthwise. Cut each piece into ½-inch-thick slices. Place slices in single layer between paper towels to remove excess moisture.

2. In 12-inch nonstick skillet, heat 1 inch water to boiling on high. Add linguine and cook as label directs. Drain and rinse under cold running water to prevent pasta from sticking.

3. In same skillet, heat 1 tablespoon oil on medium 1 minute. Add tofu in single layer and cook 10 minutes or until golden brown, turning once. Transfer to plate.

4. In same skillet, heat remaining tablespoon oil on medium 1 minute. Add celery, pepper, and garlic; cook 2 minutes or until crisp-tender, stirring. Add zucchini; cook 1 to 2 minutes or until crisp-tender, stirring.

5. Add carrots, soy sauce, tofu, chicken, and noodles. Cook 2 minutes or until heated through, stirring to coat.

6. Remove from heat, stir in sesame oil, and transfer to serving plates. Garnish with cilantro. Serve with additional soy sauce on the side, if desired.

Nutrition Facts

Each serving about:

Calories	508	Total fat	14 g	Vitamin C	59 mg
Protein	37 g	Saturated fat	2 g	Calcium	418 mg
Carbohydrate	59 g	Cholesterol	49 mg	Fiber	11 g
		Sodium	538 mg	Omega-3	10 mg

Chicken Parm Stacks

Total time 30 minutes · **Makes** 4 servings

1 slice whole wheat bread

1 teaspoon plus 1 tablespoon olive oil

¼ cup packed fresh flat-leaf parsley leaves

1 clove garlic

Salt and pepper

1 pound chicken-breast cutlets

1 pound yellow squash, cut into ½-inch-thick slices

1 pound ripe tomatoes, cut into ½-inch-thick slices

1 ounce Parmesan cheese

Basil leaves, for garnish

1. Arrange oven rack 6 inches from broiler heat source. Preheat broiler. Line 18" by 12" jelly-roll pan with foil. Preheat large ridged grill pan or prepare outdoor grill for direct grilling on medium-high.

2. In food processor with knife blade attached, pulse bread into fine crumbs. In small bowl, combine bread crumbs with 1 teaspoon oil.

3. To processor, add parsley, garlic, ¼ teaspoon each salt and freshly ground black pepper, and 1 tablespoon oil. Pulse until finely chopped.

4. On plate, rub half of parsley mixture all over chicken. Add chicken to hot grill; cook 4 minutes. Turn chicken over and cook 3 to 4 minutes longer or until 165°F and no longer pink in center.

5. Meanwhile, in prepared pan, toss squash with remaining parsley mixture; arrange in single layer. Broil 7 to 9 minutes or until squash is browned. Transfer squash to platter in single layer. Place chicken on top.

6. In same pan, arrange tomato slices in single layer. Divide crumb mixture evenly among tomatoes. Sprinkle with ⅛ teaspoon each salt and freshly ground black pepper. Broil 30 seconds or until crumbs are golden brown.

7. Arrange crumb-topped tomato slices on top of chicken. With vegetable peeler, shave Parmesan over tomatoes. Garnish with basil leaves.

SIDE FOR ONE Heat 1 cup each cooked whole-grain spaghetti and fresh spinach and ¼ cup marinara sauce until spinach is wilted.

Nutrition Facts

Each serving about:

Calories	492	Total fat	12 g	Vitamin C	30 mg
Protein	38 g	Saturated fat	3 g	Calcium	197 mg
Carbohydrate	61 g	Cholesterol	70 mg	Fiber	13 g
		Sodium	732 mg	Omega-3	210 mg

Chicken & Veggie Stir-Fry

Total time 22 minutes · **Makes** 4 servings

1½ **teaspoons olive oil**

1 **large yellow pepper, thinly sliced**

2 **cups (from 10-ounce package) shredded or matchstick carrots**

1 **pound skinless, boneless chicken-breast halves, cut into ½-inch pieces**

2 **teaspoons minced peeled fresh ginger**

2 **cloves garlic, finely chopped**

1 **package (8.8 ounces) precooked brown rice**

1¼ **cups precooked shelled edamame (thawed, if frozen)**

⅓ **cup stir-fry sauce**

3 **green onions, sliced**

⅓ **cup slivered almonds, toasted**

1. In nonstick 12-inch skillet, heat olive oil over medium-high heat until hot. Add yellow pepper and carrots and cook 2 minutes, stirring occasionally. Add chicken pieces, ginger, and garlic and cook 4 minutes, stirring constantly.

2. Add brown rice, edamame, and stir-fry sauce and cook 2 to 3 minutes longer or until chicken is no longer pink in center and rice mixture is heated through, stirring occasionally. Stir in green onions and almonds, then divide among 4 bowls to serve.

SIDE FOR ONE 1 mandarin orange.

Nutrition Facts
Each serving about:

Calories	486	Total fat	14 g	Vitamin C	116 mg
		Saturated fat	2 g	Calcium	146 mg
Protein	36 g	Cholesterol	73 mg	Fiber	6 g
Carbohydrate	52 g	Sodium	977 mg	Omega-3	60 mg

Curried Chicken Salad

Total time 35 minutes · **Makes** 4 servings

1½ pounds skinless, boneless chicken-breast halves
1 medium onion, cut into quarters
Salt
¼ cup plain nonfat yogurt
¼ cup light mayonnaise
1 tablespoon fresh lime juice
1½ teaspoons curry powder
1 teaspoon grated peeled fresh ginger
1¼ cups seedless red grapes, each cut in half
2 stalks celery, thinly sliced
1 bag (10 ounces) romaine hearts, chopped

1. Place chicken breasts in deep 12-inch skillet. Add onion quarters, ¼ teaspoon salt, and enough water to cover chicken; heat to boiling on high. Remove skillet from heat; cover and let chicken sit in poaching liquid 20 minutes. Check that it is 165°F and has lost its pink color. Transfer chicken to cutting board; cool until easy to handle.

2. Meanwhile, in large bowl, whisk yogurt, mayonnaise, lime juice, curry powder, ginger, and ¼ teaspoon salt until blended. Stir in grapes and celery.

3. Cut chicken into ½-inch chunks and add to mixture in bowl; toss to coat. Serve salad right away, or cover and refrigerate to serve chilled. Spoon chicken salad onto romaine to serve.

SIDE FOR ONE 10 Triscuit Thin Crisps or small whole-grain crackers of your choice.

DESSERT FOR ONE 1 scoop (½ cup) no-sugar-added frozen yogurt, flavor of your choice (100 calories).

Nutrition Facts

Each serving about:

Calories	502	Total fat	13 g	Vitamin C	25 mg
		Saturated fat	3 g	Calcium	247 mg
Protein	48 g	Cholesterol	114 mg	Fiber	6 g
Carbohydrate	47 g	Sodium	652 mg	Omega-3	100 mg

Fajitas Two Ways

Total time 25 minutes · **Makes** 4 servings

- 2 cloves garlic, crushed with press
- 1 teaspoon ancho chile powder
- 1 tablespoon vegetable oil
- Salt and pepper
- 12 ounces skinless, boneless chicken-breast halves
- 8 ounces beef sirloin strip steak
- 1 medium (8- to 10-ounce) onion
- 1 large (8- to 10-ounce) green bell pepper
- 1 pound red cabbage
- ½ cup packed fresh cilantro leaves
- ¼ cup reduced-fat sour cream
- 3 tablespoons fresh lime juice, plus additional lime wedges for serving
- 8 soft taco–size whole wheat flour tortillas
- Salsa, for serving

1. Arrange oven rack 6 inches from broiler heat source. Preheat broiler. Line 18" by 12" jelly-roll pan with foil.

2. In large bowl, combine garlic, chile powder, oil, and ¼ teaspoon each salt and freshly ground black pepper. Place chicken and steak in prepared pan; rub both with half of garlic mixture. Broil 8 to 10 minutes or until 165°F and juices run clear when thickest part of chicken is pierced with knife.

3. While meat cooks, thinly slice onion and bell pepper and add to bowl with remaining garlic mixture. Toss to coat. Transfer meat to cutting board and spread onion mixture in same pan. Broil 8 minutes or until vegetables are browned and tender.

4. Meanwhile, very thinly slice cabbage and chop cilantro. Transfer to large bowl. Add sour cream and lime juice and toss to coat. Thinly slice chicken and steak across grain; arrange on serving platter.

5. On large microwave-safe plate, wrap tortillas in damp paper towels and microwave on High 1 minute or until warm and pliable. Place onion mixture on serving plate and salsa and lime wedges in serving bowls. Arrange tortillas, meat, onion mixture, cabbage slaw, salsa, and limes for a do-it-yourself fajita bar.

Nutrition Facts

Each serving about:					
Calories	479	Total fat	18 g	Vitamin C	108 mg
Protein	39 g	Saturated fat	5 g	Calcium	120 mg
Carbohydrate	39 g	Cholesterol	88 mg	Fiber	6 g
		Sodium	300 mg	Omega-3	180 mg

Healthy-Makeover Meatloaf

Active time 20 minutes · **Total time** 1 hour 15 minutes · **Makes** 6 servings

1 tablespoon olive oil

2 stalks celery, finely chopped

1 small onion, finely chopped

1 clove garlic, crushed with press

2 pounds lean ground turkey

¾ cup fresh whole wheat bread crumbs (from 1½ slices bread)

⅓ cup fat-free milk

1 tablespoon Worcestershire sauce

2 large egg whites

½ cup ketchup

Salt and pepper

1 tablespoon Dijon mustard

1. Preheat oven to 350°F. In 12-inch nonstick skillet, in oil, cook celery and onion on medium 10 minutes, stirring occasionally. Add garlic and cook 1 minute. Transfer vegetables to bowl; cool slightly.

2. To bowl with vegetables, add turkey, bread crumbs, milk, Worcestershire sauce, egg whites, ¼ cup ketchup, ½ teaspoon salt, and ¼ teaspoon freshly ground black pepper; mix with hands until well combined but not overmixed. In cup, mix Dijon and remaining ¼ cup ketchup.

3. In 13" by 9" metal baking pan, shape meat mixture into 9" by 5" loaf. Spread ketchup mixture over top of loaf.

4. Bake meatloaf 55 to 60 minutes or until meat thermometer inserted in center reaches 160°F. (Temperature will rise to 165°F upon standing.)

5. Let meatloaf stand 10 minutes before removing from pan to set juices for easier slicing. Transfer meatloaf to platter and cut into slices to serve.

SIDE FOR ONE 1 cup Imagine Creamy Portobello Mushroom Soup or other mushroom soup (80 calories) garnished with 1 teaspoon minced fresh chives or ½ teaspoon dried chives. Serve ½ cup steamed green beans topped with 1 tablespoon grated Parmesan cheese alongside meatloaf.

DESSERT FOR ONE ½-cup scoop Edy's Slow Churned No Sugar Added Ice Cream, vanilla flavor, topped with 1½ teaspoons no-sugar-added blueberry jam (110 calories).

Nutrition Facts

Each serving about:

Calories	481	Total fat	16 g	Vitamin C	7 mg
Protein	47 g	Saturated fat	6 g	Calcium	389 mg
Carbohydrate	43 g	Cholesterol	100 mg	Fiber	5 g
		Sodium	1,311 mg	Omega-3	10 mg

Lemon-Mint Chicken Cutlets on Watercress

Total time 19 minutes · **Makes** 4 servings

1¼ pounds boneless, skinless chicken breasts, thinly sliced

2 lemons

2 tablespoons olive oil

2 tablespoons fresh mint, chopped

Salt and pepper

1 bag (4 ounces) baby watercress

1. Heat ridged grill pan over medium-high heat (or prepare outdoor grill for direct grilling over medium-high heat).

2. Pound chicken to uniform ¼-inch thickness if necessary.

3. From lemons, grate 1 tablespoon plus 1½ teaspoons peel and squeeze 3 tablespoons juice. In large bowl, whisk lemon peel and juice, oil, 2 tablespoons mint, ½ teaspoon salt, and ½ teaspoon freshly ground black pepper until dressing is blended.

4. Reserve ¼ cup dressing. In large bowl, toss chicken cutlets with remaining dressing. Place chicken in grill pan and cook 4 to 5 minutes or until 165°F and juices run clear when breast is pierced with tip of knife, turning over once.

5. To serve, toss watercress with reserved dressing and top with chicken. Sprinkle with additional chopped mint for garnish.

SIDE FOR ONE Mix ¾ cup Uncle Ben's Ready Rice brown rice with 1 teaspoon extra virgin olive oil; ½ teaspoon grated lemon peel; 1 green onion, minced; 1 teaspoon toasted pine nuts; and ⅛ teaspoon salt.

SALAD FOR ONE Chop ¼ cucumber and halve 6 cherry tomatoes; toss with ½ teaspoon each lemon juice and extra virgin olive oil and freshly ground black pepper to taste.

Nutrition Facts

Each serving about:					
Calories	498	Total fat	21 g	Vitamin C	44 mg
Protein	35 g	Saturated fat	3 g	Calcium	97 mg
Carbohydrate	36 g	Cholesterol	78 mg	Fiber	5 g
		Sodium	680 mg	Omega-3	180 mg

Lemon-Oregano Chicken Cutlets with Mint Zucchini

Total time 27 minutes · **Makes** 4 servings

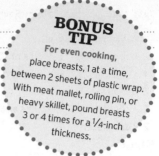

BONUS TIP
For even cooking, place breasts, 1 at a time, between 2 sheets of plastic wrap. With meat mallet, rolling pin, or heavy skillet, pound breasts 3 or 4 times for a ¼-inch thickness.

- 3 **medium zucchini (8 ounces each)**
- 2 **tablespoons olive oil**
- **Salt and pepper**
- ½ **cup loosely packed chopped fresh mint leaves**
- 4 **medium skinless, boneless chicken-breast halves (6 ounces each)**
- 3 **lemons**
- 1 **tablespoon chopped fresh oregano leaves**

1. Prepare outdoor grill for covered direct grilling on medium.

2. With mandoline or sharp knife, thinly slice zucchini lengthwise. In bowl, toss zucchini with 1 tablespoon oil, ¼ teaspoon salt, and half of mint.

3. Pound chicken breasts to uniform ¼-inch thickness. From 2 lemons, grate 1 tablespoon peel and squeeze 2 tablespoons juice. Cut remaining lemon into 4 wedges; set aside. In medium bowl, combine lemon peel and juice with oregano, remaining 1 tablespoon oil, ¼ teaspoon salt, and ½ teaspoon freshly ground black pepper; add chicken and toss.

4. Place zucchini slices, in batches, on hot grill grate and cook 2 to 4 minutes until zucchini is tender, turning over once. Remove zucchini from grill; place on large platter and sprinkle with remaining mint.

5. Place chicken on hot grill grate. Cover grill and cook chicken 6 to 8 minutes or until 165°F and juices run clear when chicken is pierced with tip of knife, turning once. Transfer chicken to platter with zucchini; serve with lemon wedges.

SIDE FOR ONE Brush 1 large whole-grain pita with ½ teaspoon extra virgin olive oil and lightly grill. Serve with 3 tablespoons tzatziki sauce.

Nutrition Facts
Each serving about:

Calories	519	Total fat	18 g	Vitamin C	42 mg
Protein	45 g	Saturated fat	4 g	Calcium	118 mg
Carbohydrate	47 g	Cholesterol	101 mg	Fiber	8 g
		Sodium	910 mg	Omega-3	320 mg

Turkey-Escarole Soup

Total time 35 minutes · **Makes** 5 servings

- 1 **tablespoon olive oil**
- 2 **cups (about two-thirds of 10-ounce bag) shredded or matchstick carrots**
- 1 **small onion, finely chopped**
- 2 **cloves garlic, minced**
- 3 **cans (14 to 14½ ounces each) low-sodium chicken broth (5¼ cups)**
- 2 **cups water**

Pepper

- 2 **heads (1½ pounds) escarole, cut into 1-inch pieces**
- ½ **cup whole wheat orzo pasta**
- 2 **cups (10 ounces) chopped leftover cooked turkey or rotisserie chicken breast**
- ½ **cup freshly grated Parmesan cheese**

1. In 6-quart Dutch oven, heat oil on medium-high until hot. Add carrots, onion, and garlic; cook 4 minutes or until onion softens, stirring frequently. Stir in broth and water; heat to boiling. Stir in escarole and orzo; heat to boiling.

2. Reduce heat to medium-low; simmer, uncovered, 6 minutes or until escarole and orzo are tender. Stir in turkey and ⅛ teaspoon freshly ground black pepper. Reduce heat to low and simmer 3 minutes until turkey is heated through. Adjust seasoning. Serve with Parmesan. Makes 10 cups.

DESSERT FOR ONE 5 dried Black Mission figs, halved; 4 walnut halves; and 4 (¼-ounce) cubes Parmesan cheese drizzled with 1½ teaspoons balsamic vinegar.

Nutrition Facts

Each serving about:					
Calories	508	Total fat	20 g	Vitamin C	13 mg
Protein	32 g	Saturated fat	8 g	Calcium	597 mg
Carbohydrate	54 g	Cholesterol	47 mg	Fiber	12 g
		Sodium	1,447 mg	Omega-3	870 mg

Turkey-Feta Burgers

Total time 25 minutes · **Makes** 4 servings

½ cup plus 2 tablespoons plain fat-free yogurt

2 teaspoons extra virgin olive oil

2 green onions, green and white parts separated and thinly sliced

½ cup packed finely chopped fresh mint leaves

1 pound lean ground turkey

1½ ounces feta cheese, finely crumbled

1½ teaspoons ground coriander

Salt and pepper

4 whole wheat pitas

2 tomatoes, thinly sliced

2 cups shredded romaine lettuce

1. Prepare outdoor grill for covered direct grilling on medium.

2. In small bowl, whisk together ½ cup yogurt and oil. Stir in white parts of green onions and half of chopped mint.

3. In large bowl, with hands, combine turkey, feta, coriander, ⅛ teaspoon each salt and freshly ground black pepper, green parts of green onions, remaining mint, and remaining yogurt. Mix well, then form into four 4½-inch round patties (each about ½ inch thick).

4. Place patties on hot grill grate; cover and cook 10 to 12 minutes or until meat loses its pink color throughout, turning once. (Burgers should reach an internal temperature of 160°F.) During last 2 minutes of cooking, warm pitas on grill, turning once. Sprinkle with ⅛ teaspoon freshly ground black pepper.

5. Open pitas. Divide burgers, tomato slices, lettuce, and yogurt sauce among pitas.

SIDE FOR ONE 1 bunch red or black seedless grapes (20 grapes).

Nutrition Facts
Each serving about:

Calories	480	Total fat	16 g	Vitamin C	11 mg
Protein	31 g	Saturated fat	5 g	Calcium	168 mg
Carbohydrate	59 g	Cholesterol	100 mg	Fiber	6 g
		Sodium	599 mg	Omega-3	230 mg

Orange Pork & Asparagus Stir-Fry

Active time 20 minutes · **Total time** 26 minutes · **Makes** 4 servings

> 2 navel oranges
>
> 1 teaspoon peanut or olive oil
>
> 1 whole pork tenderloin (about ¾ pound), trimmed and thinly sliced diagonally
>
> Salt and pepper
>
> 1½ pounds thin asparagus, trimmed, each stalk cut crosswise in half
>
> 1 clove garlic, crushed with press
>
> ¼ cup water
>
> ⅓ cup roasted unsalted cashews or peanuts, chopped

1. From 1 orange, grate 1 teaspoon peel and squeeze ¼ cup juice. Remove peel and white pith from remaining orange. Cut orange into ¼-inch-thick slices; cut each slice into quarters.

2. In nonstick 12-inch skillet, heat ½ teaspoon oil over medium-high heat until hot but not smoking. Add half of pork and sprinkle with ¼ teaspoon salt and ⅛ teaspoon freshly ground black pepper; cook, stirring frequently (stir-frying), until pork just loses its pink color, about 2 minutes. Transfer pork to plate. Repeat with remaining pork, again using ½ teaspoon oil, ¼ teaspoon salt, and ⅛ teaspoon pepper. Transfer pork to same plate.

3. To same skillet, add asparagus, garlic, grated orange peel, ¼ teaspoon salt, and water; cover and cook, stirring occasionally, until asparagus is tender-crisp, about 2 minutes. Return pork to skillet. Add reserved orange juice and orange pieces; heat through, stirring often. Sprinkle with cashews.

SIDE FOR ONE Mix 1 cup cooked whole wheat couscous with 2 green onions, minced; 1 tablespoon chopped fresh cilantro (optional); 8 roasted cashews or 12 peanuts, chopped; 1 teaspoon peanut oil; ½ teaspoon grated orange peel; and ⅛ teaspoon salt.

Nutrition Facts
Each serving about:

Calories	489	Total fat	14 g	Vitamin C	41 mg
Protein	32 g	Saturated fat	3 g	Calcium	101 mg
Carbohydrate	65 g	Cholesterol	55 mg	Fiber	12 g
		Sodium	781 mg	Omega-3	40 mg

Pulled Pork on a Bun

Total time 30 minutes · **Makes** 4 servings

- 1 **tablespoon water**
- 1½ **teaspoons salt-free chili powder**
- 1 **teaspoon smoked paprika**
- 1 **teaspoon dry mustard powder**
- **Salt and pepper**
- 1 **pound pork tenderloin,**
  cut into 2-inch-thick medallions
- 3 **cups shredded cabbage mix**
  for coleslaw

- 2 **tablespoons plus 1 teaspoon**
  apple cider vinegar
- 2 **tablespoons snipped fresh chives**
- 1 **tablespoon plus 2 teaspoons**
  spicy brown mustard
- ⅓ **cup barbecue sauce**
  (preferably no-sugar-added)
- 4 **soft whole wheat hamburger buns,**
  lightly toasted

1. Fill 6-quart saucepot with 1 inch water and add steamer insert. Cover; heat to boiling on high. Reduce heat to medium.

2. In small bowl, combine chili powder, smoked paprika, dry mustard, ¼ teaspoon salt, and ¼ teaspoon freshly ground black pepper. Rub spices all over pork. Place pork in steamer; cover and steam 18 to 20 minutes or until pork is 145°F in center, turning over once.

3. Meanwhile, in medium bowl, toss cabbage mix with 2 tablespoons vinegar, chives, 1 tablespoon mustard, and ⅛ teaspoon salt; set aside.

4. Transfer pork to plate. Discard water in pot; remove steamer. When cool enough to handle, shred pork into bite-size pieces.

5. Return pork to saucepot. Stir in barbecue sauce, 1 tablespoon water, and remaining 2 teaspoons mustard and 1 teaspoon vinegar. Cook on medium until hot, stirring frequently. Divide pork and slaw among buns.

SIDE FOR ONE 15 SunChips, Original or Harvest Cheddar flavor (120 calories).

DESSERT FOR ONE 1 wedge watermelon or 1 cup fresh pineapple chunks.

Nutrition Facts

Each serving about:

Calories	513	Total fat	12 g	Vitamin C	43 mg
Protein	31 g	Saturated fat	2 g	Calcium	106 mg
Carbohydrate	73 g	Cholesterol	62 mg	Fiber	8 g
		Sodium	779 mg	Omega-3	90 mg

Spice-Rubbed Pork Tenderloin

Active time 5 minutes · **Total time** 25 minutes · **Makes** 4 servings

  1 **tablespoon curry powder**
  1 **teaspoon ground cumin**
Salt
  ¼ **teaspoon ground cinnamon**
  2 **teaspoons vegetable oil**
  1 **(1-pound) pork tenderloin**

1. Preheat broiler. In cup, combine curry powder, cumin, ¾ teaspoon salt, cinnamon, and oil; use to rub on tenderloin.

2. Place tenderloin on rack in broiling pan. Place pan in broiler 5 to 7 inches from heat source. Broil tenderloin, turning once, until meat thermometer inserted in center of pork reaches 145°F, 14 to 18 minutes. (Internal temperature will rise to 150°F upon standing.)

3. Place meat on cutting board. Let stand 5 minutes to set juices for easier slicing. With knife held in slanted position, almost parallel to board, cut tenderloin into ¼-inch-thick slices.

SIDE FOR ONE Stir together 1 cup Uncle Ben's Ready Rice brown rice with 1 small yellow summer squash or zucchini, diced and steamed (about 1 cup), 2 tablespoons toasted pine nuts or sliced natural almonds, 1 teaspoon extra virgin olive oil, and ⅛ teaspoon salt; garnish with fresh cilantro leaves, if desired.

Nutrition Facts

Each serving about:					
Calories	485	Total fat	20 g	Vitamin C	7 mg
Protein	32 g	Saturated fat	3 g	Calcium	82 mg
Carbohydrate	48 g	Cholesterol	74 mg	Fiber	7 g
		Sodium	804 mg	Omega-3	160 mg

Beef Ragu

Total time 30 minutes · **Makes** 6 servings

Salt and pepper

2 teaspoons extra virgin olive oil

1 pound lean (93%) ground beef

1 large carrot, finely chopped

1 large stalk celery, finely chopped

1 small (4- to 6-ounce) onion, finely chopped

¼ teaspoon ground cumin

¼ teaspoon ground coriander

1 pinch crushed red pepper

1 can (14½ ounces) no-salt-added fire-roasted diced tomatoes

1 package (13¼ ounces) whole-grain penne

1 cup packed fresh mint leaves, finely chopped

½ cup goat cheese, crumbled

1. Heat covered 6-quart pot of water to boiling on high. Add 2 teaspoons salt.

2. In 12-inch skillet, heat oil on high. Add beef in even layer. Sprinkle with ¼ teaspoon each salt and freshly ground black pepper. Cook 2 minutes or until browned; stir, breaking into pieces.

3. Add carrot, celery, and onion. Cook 5 minutes or until tender and golden, stirring occasionally. Add cumin, coriander, and red pepper. Cook 30 seconds, stirring. Stir in tomatoes; heat to boiling. Reduce heat to maintain steady simmer. Simmer 10 minutes.

4. Meanwhile, add penne to boiling water. Cook 1 minute less than minimum time label directs. Drain, reserving ½ cup pasta cooking water. Return pasta to saucepot. Stir in tomato sauce and reserved pasta cooking water; cook on medium 2 minutes or until pasta is al dente and well coated, stirring. Stir in mint and ¼ teaspoon each salt and freshly ground black pepper and top with crumbled goat cheese.

DESSERT FOR ONE 1 peach or nectarine, sliced.

Nutrition Facts
Each serving about:

Calories	484	Total fat	12 g	Vitamin C	25 mg
Protein	30 g	Saturated fat	5 g	Calcium	119 mg
Carbohydrate	70 g	Cholesterol	56 mg	Fiber	10 g
		Sodium	408 mg	Omega-3	100 mg

Steak & Oven Fries

Total time 30 minutes · **Makes** 4 servings

Oven Fries

　3 **unpeeled baking potatoes (8 ounces each)**
　3 **teaspoons olive oil**
Salt and pepper

Steak

1¼ **pounds beef flank steak, trimmed of fat**
½ **teaspoon dried tarragon**
　1 **medium shallot, minced**
¾ **cup dry red wine**
　1 **bag (9 ounces) microwave-in-the-bag baby spinach**

1. Prepare Oven Fries: Preheat oven to 450°F. Cut each unpeeled potato crosswise in half, then cut each half lengthwise into 8 wedges.

2. Spray 15½" by 10½" jelly-roll pan or 2 large cookie sheets with nonstick cooking spray. Place potatoes in pan and toss with 2 teaspoons oil and ¼ teaspoon each salt and freshly ground black pepper. Roast potatoes in oven 25 minutes or until fork-tender and beginning to brown, stirring once halfway through roasting.

3. Prepare Steak: While Oven Fries are cooking, rub steak on both sides with tarragon and ¼ teaspoon salt. Heat 12-inch cast-iron or other heavy skillet over medium-high heat until hot. Add 1 teaspoon oil and steak; cook 12 minutes for medium (145°F), or until desired doneness, turning over once. Remove steak to cutting board; keep warm.

4. To same skillet, add shallot and cook 1 minute, stirring. Add red wine and heat to boiling; boil 2 minutes or until reduced to ⅓ cup.

5. Cook spinach in microwave as label directs. Thinly slice steak and serve with wine sauce, potatoes, and spinach.

SIDE FOR ONE 1 cup cherries or ¾ cup grapes.

Nutrition Facts

Each serving about:

Calories	527	Total fat	14 g	Vitamin C	24 mg
Protein	37 g	Saturated fat	4 g	Calcium	132 mg
Carbohydrate	61 g	Cholesterol	60 mg	Fiber	8 g
		Sodium	366 mg	Omega-3	110 mg

Steak Sandwich with Grilled Onions

Total time 27 minutes · **Makes** 4 servings

¼ **cup soy sauce**

¼ **cup balsamic vinegar**

1 **tablespoon brown sugar (optional)**

1 **teaspoon fresh thyme leaves**

Pepper

1 **(1¼-pound) beef flank steak**

1 **medium (8-ounce) red onion, cut into 4 thick slices**

8 **slices whole-grain sourdough bread, toasted on grill if you like**

2 **medium ripe tomatoes, sliced**

1 **bunch arugula, tough stems discarded**

1. In large self-sealing plastic bag, mix soy sauce, vinegar, sugar (if using), thyme, and ¼ teaspoon freshly ground black pepper. Add steak to marinade, turning to coat. Seal bag, pressing out excess air. Place bag on plate; let stand 15 minutes at room temperature or 1 hour in the refrigerator, turning over several times.

2. Meanwhile, for easier handling, insert 1 long metal skewer horizontally through onion slices; set aside. Prepare charcoal fire or preheat gas grill for covered direct grilling over medium heat.

3. Remove steak from marinade; pour marinade into 1-quart saucepan. Heat marinade over high heat to boiling; boil 2 minutes.

4. Place steak and onion slices on hot grill grate. Cover grill and cook steak and onion 12 to 15 minutes or until onion is browned and tender and meat is medium (145°F), brushing both with marinade occasionally and turning both over once. Transfer steak to cutting board; separate onion into rings.

5. Thinly slice steak diagonally across the grain. Arrange onion rings and steak on 4 slices of bread; spoon any meat juices from board over onion and steak. Top with tomatoes, arugula, and remaining 4 slices of bread.

DESSERT FOR ONE 1 small banana, unpeeled, halved lengthwise, with cut surfaces spritzed with cooking spray and grilled until grill marks have formed as desired. (Remove peel before eating.)

Nutrition Facts

Each serving about:

Calories	522	Total fat	10 g	Vitamin C	23 mg
		Saturated fat	3 g	Calcium	104 mg
Protein	40 g	Cholesterol	47 mg	Fiber	8 g
Carbohydrate	64 g	Sodium	988 mg	Omega-3	100 mg

Almond-Crusted Tilapia

Total time 30 minutes · **Makes** 4 servings

2 lemons

2 tablespoons olive oil

Salt and pepper

4 tilapia fillets (6 ounces each)

¼ cup sliced natural almonds

1 small onion, chopped

1 bag (12 ounces) trimmed fresh green beans

1 package (10 ounces) sliced white mushrooms

2 tablespoons water

1. Preheat oven to 425°F. From 1 lemon, grate 1 teaspoon peel and squeeze 3 tablespoons juice; cut second lemon into wedges. In cup, mix lemon peel and 1 tablespoon juice, 1 tablespoon oil, ¼ teaspoon salt, and ⅛ teaspoon freshly ground black pepper.

2. Spray 13" by 9" glass baking dish with nonstick spray; place tilapia, dark side down, in dish. Drizzle tilapia with lemon mixture; top with almonds, pressing them on. Bake 15 minutes or until tilapia turns opaque.

3. Meanwhile, in 12-inch skillet, heat remaining 1 tablespoon oil on medium-high 1 minute. Add onion and cook 5 to 6 minutes or until golden, stirring occasionally. Stir in green beans, mushrooms, water, ¼ teaspoon salt, and ⅛ teaspoon freshly ground black pepper. Cook about 6 minutes or until most of liquid evaporates and green beans are tender-crisp. Toss with remaining 2 tablespoons lemon juice. Serve bean mixture and lemon wedges with tilapia.

SIDE FOR ONE Sprinkle ¼ cup cooked whole wheat orzo with ¼ teaspoon extra virgin olive oil, 1 teaspoon Pecorino Romano cheese, and freshly cracked black peppercorns to taste.

DESSERT FOR ONE Toss 1 cup sliced strawberries with 1 teaspoon lemon juice and thinly sliced fresh basil to taste (optional).

Nutrition Facts

Each serving about:					
Calories	494	Total fat	15 g	Vitamin C	125 mg
Protein	46 g	Saturated fat	3 g	Calcium	139 mg
Carbohydrate	49 g	Cholesterol	88 mg	Fiber	12 g
		Sodium	145 mg	Omega-3	430 mg

Chipotle-Orange–Glazed Salmon

Total time 40 minutes · **Makes** 4 servings

1 cup quinoa, rinsed

1 orange

1 chipotle chile in adobo sauce

2 teaspoons adobo sauce (from chipotle chiles)

1 clove garlic, peeled

½ teaspoon ground cumin

1 bunch radishes, trimmed, halved, and thinly sliced

1 cup fresh corn kernels (from 2 ears)

½ cup fresh cilantro leaves, chopped

2 green onions, sliced

Salt

4 pieces skinless salmon fillet (5 ounces each)

3 tablespoons sliced natural almonds, toasted

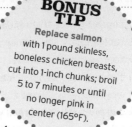

BONUS TIP

Replace salmon with 1 pound skinless, boneless chicken breasts, cut into 1-inch chunks; broil 5 to 7 minutes or until no longer pink in center (165°F).

1. Arrange oven rack 4 to 6 inches from broiler heat source. Preheat broiler on high. Line 15½" by 10½" jelly-roll pan with foil. In 2-quart saucepan, prepare quinoa as label directs. Transfer to bowl.

2. Meanwhile, from orange, grate 1 teaspoon peel and squeeze ½ cup juice. In blender, puree chipotle, adobo sauce, garlic, cumin, and orange juice.

3. To bowl with quinoa, stir in radishes, corn, cilantro, green onions, orange peel, and ⅛ teaspoon salt.

4. Arrange salmon on prepared pan. Sprinkle with ⅛ teaspoon salt, then brush generously on all sides with chile mixture. Broil 5 to 7 minutes or until just opaque throughout. Serve salmon on quinoa pilaf. Sprinkle with almonds.

SIDE FOR ONE Toss ¼ avocado, cut into chunks, with 5 grape tomatoes, halved. Sprinkle with balsamic vinegar.

Nutrition Facts
Each serving about:

Calories	476	Total fat	16 g	Vitamin C 38 mg
Protein	38 g	Saturated fat	3 g	Calcium 119 mg
Carbohydrate	46 g	Cholesterol	66 mg	Fiber 8 g
		Sodium	250 mg	Omega-3 1,580 mg

Crispy Fish Sandwiches

Total time 15 minutes · **Makes** 4 servings

3 cups (6 ounces) shredded red cabbage

2 tablespoons apple cider vinegar

½ teaspoon celery seeds

¼ cup packed fresh flat-leaf parsley leaves, finely chopped

¼ cup plain fat-free Greek yogurt

2 tablespoons mayonnaise

2 tablespoons sweet pickle relish

1 tablespoon fresh lemon juice

1 teaspoon Dijon mustard

Salt and pepper

2 large egg whites

¾ cup plain dried whole wheat bread crumbs

4 skinless flounder fillets (4 ounces each)

4 whole wheat hamburger buns, toasted

½ seedless (English) cucumber, very thinly sliced

1. Arrange oven rack 4 inches from heat source. Preheat broiler on high. Lightly coat 18" by 12" jelly-roll pan with nonstick cooking spray.

2. In large bowl, combine cabbage, vinegar, and celery seeds; toss well. Set aside. In small bowl, with wire whisk, stir together parsley, yogurt, mayonnaise, relish, lemon juice, mustard, and ⅛ teaspoon each salt and freshly ground black pepper; cover and refrigerate.

3. In pie plate, whisk egg whites with fork just until frothy. Place crumbs on waxed paper. Season flounder with ¼ teaspoon each salt and freshly ground black pepper. Dip flounder into egg whites, then coat with crumbs, patting to cover both sides. Arrange on prepared pan. Broil 2½ to 3 minutes or until golden brown on both sides, turning once.

4. Cut each fillet in half. Spread 2 tablespoons tartar sauce on bottom of each bun; top with cucumber, 2 pieces flounder, and ¾ cup slaw. Replace tops of buns to serve.

SIDE FOR ONE Toss 2 cups lettuce with ¼ medium apple, diced; 1 tablespoon chopped roasted walnuts; 1 teaspoon canola oil; and apple cider vinegar to taste. Sprinkle with 2 teaspoons crumbled blue cheese.

Nutrition Facts

Each serving about:					
Calories	502	Total fat	21 g	Vitamin C	46 mg
Protein	27 g	Saturated fat	4 g	Calcium	191 mg
Carbohydrate	55 g	Cholesterol	51 mg	Fiber	10 g
		Sodium	1,043 mg	Omega-3	3,540 mg

Fresh Salmon Burgers with Capers & Dill

Total time 31 minutes · **Makes** 4 servings

1 large lemon

¼ cup light mayonnaise

1 tablespoon capers, drained and coarsely chopped

1 (1-pound) salmon fillet, skin removed

¼ cup loosely packed chopped fresh dill

2 green onions, thinly sliced

½ cup plain dried whole wheat or other whole-grain bread crumbs

Salt

Nonstick cooking spray

4 whole wheat or other whole-grain hamburger buns, split and toasted

Green-leaf lettuce leaves

1. Prepare outdoor grill for direct grilling over medium heat.

2. Meanwhile, from lemon, grate 1 teaspoon peel and squeeze 1 tablespoon juice.

3. In small bowl, stir lemon juice and ½ teaspoon lemon peel with mayonnaise and capers until blended. Set lemon-caper sauce aside. Makes about ⅓ cup.

4. With large chef's knife, finely chop salmon; place in medium bowl. Add dill, green onions, ¼ cup bread crumbs, ¾ teaspoon salt, and remaining ½ teaspoon lemon peel to salmon; gently mix with fork until combined. Shape salmon mixture into four 3-inch round burgers.

5. Sprinkle both sides of burgers with remaining bread crumbs. Spray both sides of burgers with nonstick spray.

6. Place burgers on hot grill rack. Cook burgers 6 to 8 minutes or until browned on the outside and still slightly pink in the center for medium or until desired doneness, turning burgers over once.

7. Serve burgers on buns with lettuce and lemon-caper mayonnaise.

SIDE FOR ONE 1 cup steamed baby carrots.

DESSERT FOR ONE 1 small apple (cut into wedges, if desired).

Nutrition Facts

Each serving about:

Calories	508	Total fat	16 g	Vitamin C	14 mg
Protein	32 g	Saturated fat	2 g	Calcium	117 mg
Carbohydrate	61 g	Cholesterol	77 mg	Fiber	12 g
		Sodium	953 mg	Omega-3	2,790 mg

Grilled Fish Tacos

Total time 20 minutes · **Makes** 6 servings

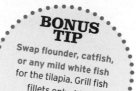

BONUS TIP

Swap flounder, catfish, or any mild white fish for the tilapia. Grill fish fillets only 4 to 5 minutes per ½ inch of thickness.

1 lemon

2½ teaspoons vegetable oil

Salt

2 ears corn, husked

1 avocado, cut in half and pitted

3 cloves garlic, crushed with press

½ teaspoon dried oregano

¼ teaspoon cayenne
   (ground red pepper)

1 pound skinless tilapia fillets

12 corn tortillas

½ large ripe tomato, finely chopped

Fresh cilantro leaves, for serving

Lime wedges, for serving

1. Prepare outdoor grill for grilling on medium-high. From lemon, grate 2 teaspoons peel and squeeze 2 tablespoons juice.

2. Rub ½ teaspoon oil and pinch salt all over corn and cut sides of avocado. On plate, mix garlic, oregano, cayenne, lemon peel, ¼ teaspoon salt, and 2 teaspoons oil; add fish and coat with mixture.

3. Place fish, corn, and avocado, cut sides down, on hot grill grate. Cook fish 3 to 4 minutes or until opaque throughout, turning over once; cook vegetables 5 minutes or until charred, turning occasionally.

4. Transfer fish, corn, and avocado to cutting board. Grill tortillas in single layer 1 minute, turning once. Stack on large sheet of foil and wrap tightly.

5. Cut kernels from cobs. Peel and chop avocado. Break fish into chunks. In bowl, mix tomato, corn, avocado, lemon juice, and ¼ teaspoon salt. Divide fish and vegetables among tortillas; serve with cilantro and lime.

BEAN SALAD FOR ONE Chop 1 large tomato and toss with ½ cup black beans and 1 teaspoon each chopped cilantro, lime juice, and canola oil.

DESSERT FOR ONE ½ cup pineapple, fresh or canned in juice (not syrup) and drained.

Nutrition Facts

Each serving about:

Calories	506	Total fat	11 g	Vitamin C	38 mg
Protein	29 g	Saturated fat	2 g	Calcium	210 mg
Carbohydrate	80 g	Cholesterol	38 mg	Fiber	15 g
		Sodium	156 mg	Omega-3	170 mg

Niçoise Salad

Total time 25 minutes • **Makes** 4 servings

4 **large eggs**

½ **pound green beans, trimmed**

2 **tablespoons white wine vinegar**

1 **tablespoon minced shallot**

1 **teaspoon Dijon mustard**

Salt and pepper

¼ **teaspoon sugar**

3 **tablespoons olive oil**

1 **package (10 ounces) European-blend salad greens**

1 **can (19 ounces) white kidney (cannellini) beans, rinsed and drained**

½ **cup (about 2 ounces) Kalamata olives, pitted**

1 **can (5 ounces) no-salt-added albacore tuna, flaked**

1. In small saucepan, hard-cook eggs.

2. Meanwhile, in 10-inch skillet, heat 1 inch water to boiling over high heat. Add green beans; heat to boiling. Reduce heat to low; simmer 5 to 8 minutes, until beans are tender. Drain beans; immediately rinse with cold running water to stop cooking.

3. In small bowl, with wire whisk, combine vinegar, shallot, Dijon, ½ teaspoon salt, ¼ teaspoon freshly ground black pepper, and sugar. Slowly whisk in olive oil until dressing thickens slightly.

4. Remove shells from eggs. Cut each egg lengthwise into quarters.

5. To serve: Into medium bowl, pour half of dressing. Add salad greens; toss to coat. Line large platter with dressed salad greens. Arrange green beans, white kidney beans, olives, egg quarters, and tuna in separate piles on top of lettuce. Drizzle remaining dressing over salad.

SIDE FOR ONE 6 slices unsalted whole-grain melba toasts or 1 (1½-ounce) rye-bread roll.

Nutrition Facts

Each serving about:

Calories	489	Total fat	20 g	Vitamin C	14 mg
Protein	24 g	Saturated fat	4 g	Calcium	111 mg
Carbohydrate	52 g	Cholesterol	198 mg	Fiber	11 g
		Sodium	783 mg	Omega-3	430 mg

Pomegranate-Glazed Salmon

Total time 30 minutes · **Makes** 4 servings

¾ cup 100% pomegranate juice (without added sugar)

¼ cup orange juice

1 cup bulgur

2 cups water

4 pieces (5 ounces each) skinless center-cut salmon fillet

Salt and pepper

5 ounces radishes

5 dried-apricot halves

3 green onions

1. Preheat oven to 450°F. Line 18" by 12" jelly-roll pan with foil.

2. In 1-quart saucepan, heat pomegranate and orange juices to boiling on high. Reduce heat to medium-low; simmer 15 minutes or until reduced to ⅓ cup.

3. In large microwave-safe bowl, combine bulgur and water. Microwave on High 10 to 12 minutes or until bulgur is tender and water is absorbed.

4. Arrange salmon in prepared pan; sprinkle with ⅛ teaspoon each salt and freshly ground black pepper. Roast 8 to 10 minutes or until fish just turns opaque.

5. Meanwhile, finely chop radishes, apricots, and green onions. Reserve 1 tablespoon green onion.

6. Add remaining green onion to bulgur along with radishes, apricots, and ⅛ teaspoon each salt and freshly ground black pepper; stir to combine. Divide among serving plates. Top with salmon, then glaze. Garnish with reserved green onion.

SIDE FOR ONE 1 cup sugar snap peas, steamed.

Nutrition Facts
Each serving about:

Calories	480	Total fat	16 g	Vitamin C	85 mg
Protein	37 g	Saturated fat	3 g	Calcium	110 mg
Carbohydrate	48 g	Cholesterol	84 mg	Fiber	11 g
		Sodium	122 mg	Omega-3	2,860 mg

Salmon with Peppers & Pilaf

Total time 30 minutes · **Makes** 4 servings

- 2 **cups quick-cooking brown rice**
- 1½ **teaspoons canola oil**
- **Salt and pepper**
- 4 **skinless center-cut salmon fillets (6 ounces each)**
- 2 **limes, 1 cut into wedges**
- 3 **small bell peppers (red, orange, and yellow)**
- 1 **medium (6- to 8-ounce) onion**
- ½ **cup packed fresh basil leaves**
- 6 **ounces baby spinach**
- 3 **tablespoons pine nuts, toasted**

1. Prepare rice as label directs.

2. In 12-inch nonstick skillet, heat ½ teaspoon oil on medium 1 minute. Sprinkle ¼ teaspoon salt and ⅛ teaspoon pepper on salmon. Add to skillet; cook 8 to 10 minutes or until opaque throughout, turning once. Transfer to serving plates. Grate peel of whole lime over fish.

3. While salmon cooks, slice peppers very thinly. Finely chop onion.

4. Drain fat from skillet. Heat 1 teaspoon oil in skillet on medium 1 minute. Add peppers, onion, 3 tablespoons water, and ⅛ teaspoon salt. Cover; cook 5 minutes. Uncover; cook 3 to 5 minutes longer or until tender, stirring occasionally. Stir in basil and cook until wilted. From lime, squeeze 1 tablespoon juice into mixture.

5. Meanwhile, in large bowl, combine spinach and pinch salt. Cover with vented plastic wrap; microwave on High 3 minutes or until wilted. Spoon next to salmon, along with rice and pepper mixture. Adjust seasoning. Sprinkle with pine nuts. Serve with lime wedges.

Nutrition Facts

Each serving about:

Calories	482	Total fat	25 g	Vitamin C	72 mg
Protein	38 g	Saturated fat	6 g	Calcium	98 mg
Carbohydrate	27 g	Cholesterol	85 mg	Fiber	6 g
		Sodium	197 mg	Omega-3	3,650 mg

Scallop & Cherry Tomato Skewers

Total time 25 minutes · **Makes** 4 servings

8 (8-inch) bamboo skewers
1 lemon
2 tablespoons olive oil
2 tablespoons Dijon mustard
Salt
24 cherry tomatoes
16 large sea scallops

1. Soak skewers in hot water at least 30 minutes. Prepare outdoor grill for direct grilling on medium.

2. Meanwhile, from lemon, grate 1½ teaspoons peel and squeeze 1 tablespoon juice. In small bowl, whisk lemon peel and juice, oil, Dijon, and ⅛ teaspoon salt until blended; set aside.

3. Thread 3 tomatoes and 2 scallops alternately on each skewer, beginning and ending with tomato.

4. Brush scallops and tomatoes with half of Dijon mixture; place on hot grill grate. Cook 7 to 9 minutes, turning several times. Brush with remaining Dijon mixture and cook 5 minutes longer or until scallops just turn opaque throughout.

SIDE FOR ONE Toss 3 cups mixed salad greens with 12 whole-grain pita chips, coarsely broken; 1 tablespoon grated Pecorino Romano cheese; 2 teaspoons extra virgin olive oil; and 1½ tablespoons red wine vinegar or to taste.

Nutrition Facts

Each serving about:					
Calories	504	Total fat	25 g	Vitamin C	43 mg
		Saturated fat	6 g	Calcium	230 mg
Protein	29 g	Cholesterol	53 mg	Fiber	8 g
Carbohydrate	41 g	Sodium	1,204 mg	Omega-3	250 mg

Seared Salmon with Sweet Potatoes

Total time 30 minutes · **Makes** 4 servings

- 1 **pound sweet potatoes, peeled and cut into ½-inch cubes**
- ½ **cup water**
- **Salt and pepper**
- 1 **bag (5 to 6 ounces) baby spinach**
- ⅛ **teaspoon cayenne pepper**
- 4 **pieces (5 ounces each) skinless center-cut salmon fillet**
- 2 **tablespoons olive oil**
- 1 **lemon**
- 1 **cup dry white wine**
- 2 **teaspoons capers, rinsed**
- ¼ **cup chopped fresh flat-leaf parsley**

1. In large microwave-safe bowl, combine potatoes, water, and ¼ teaspoon each salt and freshly ground pepper. Cover with vented plastic wrap; microwave on High 9 minutes or until tender, stirring halfway through. Add spinach; re-cover and microwave 2 minutes longer.

2. Meanwhile, sprinkle cayenne and ⅛ teaspoon salt on salmon. Heat oil in 12-inch nonstick skillet on medium. Add salmon and cook 10 minutes or until knife pierces center easily (145°F), turning over halfway through cooking. Transfer to plate. From lemon, finely grate ½ teaspoon peel onto fish; into cup, squeeze 1 tablespoon juice.

3. To skillet, add wine and capers. Boil on high 2 minutes or until liquid is reduced by half, scraping browned bits from pan. Remove from heat; stir in lemon juice and parsley.

4. Divide potato mixture among plates; top with fish. Spoon sauce over fish.

DESSERT FOR ONE 1 large orange, segmented, tossed with ¼ cup pomegranate seeds or blueberries.

Nutrition Facts
Each serving about:

Calories	478	Total fat	17 g	Vitamin C	126 mg
Protein	33 g	Saturated fat	2 g	Calcium	156 mg
Carbohydrate	51 g	Cholesterol	78 mg	Fiber	11 g
		Sodium	433 mg	Omega-3	3,040 mg

Shrimp & Fresh Corn Grits

Total time 25 minutes · **Makes** 4 servings

1 cup (1%) low-fat milk

1½ cups water

Salt

½ cup quick-cooking grits

1 teaspoon vegetable oil

1 (3-ounce) link fully cooked andouille sausage, cut into ¼-inch pieces

1 large (10- to 12-ounce) onion

1 large (10-ounce) red bell pepper, finely chopped

12 ounces (20- to 23-count) large shrimp, peeled and deveined

1 teaspoon salt-free Cajun seasoning

5 cups fresh corn kernels or frozen corn kernels, thawed

1. In 4-quart saucepan, heat milk, 1 cup water, and pinch salt to boiling. Whisk in grits, cover, and reduce heat to medium-low. Simmer 10 minutes or until tender, whisking occasionally.

2. Meanwhile, in 12-inch skillet, heat oil on medium-high. Add sausage and cook 2 minutes or until browned, stirring occasionally. Add onion, red pepper, and ⅛ teaspoon salt. Cook 5 minutes or until just tender and browned, stirring.

3. Stir in shrimp and Cajun seasoning. Cook 1 minute, stirring. Add remaining ⅓ cup water; cook 2 minutes or until shrimp just turn opaque, stirring.

4. Stir corn into grits; cook 1 minute. Serve topped with shrimp mixture.

SIDE FOR ONE ⅔ cup pineapple cubes, sprinkled with ½ teaspoon chopped fresh mint or cilantro if desired.

Nutrition Facts

Each serving about:

Calories	514	Total fat	10 g	Vitamin C	165 mg
Protein	32 g	Saturated fat	3 g	Calcium	166 mg
Carbohydrate	82 g	Cholesterol	144 mg	Fiber	10 g
		Sodium	355 mg	Omega-3	490 mg

Soba Noodle Bowl with Shrimp & Snow Peas

Active time 15 minutes · **Total time** 35 minutes · **Makes** 4 servings

¼ cup creamy peanut butter

2 teaspoons grated peeled fresh ginger

1½ tablespoons reduced-sodium soy sauce

1½ tablespoons rice vinegar or white wine vinegar

1 teaspoon Asian sesame oil

½ teaspoon hot-pepper sauce

Salt

1 package (8 ounces) 100% whole buckwheat soba noodles or whole wheat linguine

½ bag (10 ounces) shredded or matchstick carrots (1½ cups)

8 ounces large shrimp, shelled and deveined, with tail part left on if you like

4 ounces snow peas, strings removed

½ cup loosely packed fresh cilantro leaves, chopped, plus additional sprigs for garnish

½ cup unsalted dry-roasted peanuts

1. In small bowl, place peanut butter, ginger, soy sauce, vinegar, sesame oil, and hot-pepper sauce. Set aside.

2. Heat covered 5- to 6-quart saucepot of water and 1 teaspoon salt to boiling over high heat. Add noodles and cook 4 minutes (or per package directions). Add carrots and cook 1 minute. Add shrimp and snow peas and cook 2 minutes more. Reserve ½ cup noodle cooking water. Drain noodles, shrimp, and vegetables into large colander, then transfer to large bowl.

3. With wire whisk, beat peanut butter mixture until well blended. Add peanut sauce and chopped cilantro to noodle mixture in bowl and toss until evenly coated. Add peanuts and toss.

4. To serve, spoon into four large bowls; garnish each serving with a cilantro sprig.

SIDE FOR ONE 1 cup brewed chai tea with ¼ cup fat-free milk or soy milk and, if desired, zero-calorie sweetener to taste.

Nutrition Facts
Each serving about:

Calories	502	Total fat	20 g	Vitamin C	17 mg
Protein	25 g	Saturated fat	3 g	Calcium	158 mg
Carbohydrate	60 g	Cholesterol	73 mg	Fiber	7 g
		Sodium	867 mg	Omega-3	50 mg

Steamed Scrod Fillet Dinner

Active time 15 minutes · **Total time** 25 minutes · **Makes** 4 servings

- 2 tablespoons reduced-sodium soy sauce
- 2 tablespoons seasoned rice vinegar
- 2 tablespoons 100% orange or pineapple juice
- 1 tablespoon finely chopped peeled fresh ginger
- 1 clove garlic, crushed with press
- 1 pound bok choy, coarsely chopped
- 1¾ cups peeled, shredded carrots
- 4 scrod fillets (6 ounces each)
- 4 green onions, sliced
- 1 cup whole wheat couscous
- 2 teaspoons Asian toasted sesame oil
- 1 teaspoon grated orange peel (optional)
- ¾ cup sliced almonds, toasted

1. In small bowl, with fork, mix soy sauce, vinegar, juice, ginger, and garlic.

2. In 12-inch skillet, toss bok choy and carrots. Fold thin ends of scrod fillets under to create even thickness. Place scrod on top of vegetables. Pour soy-sauce mixture over scrod and sprinkle with three-quarters of green onions; cover and heat to boiling over high heat. Reduce heat to medium; cook until scrod is just opaque throughout, about 10 minutes.

3. Meanwhile, prepare couscous according to package directions. Stir in sesame oil, orange peel (if using), remaining green onions, and ½ cup almonds.

4. Serve scrod and vegetables over couscous, drizzling with all sauce from skillet. Top with remaining almonds. Serve with additional reduced-sodium soy sauce on the side, if desired.

SIDE FOR ONE 1 orange or ¾ cup pineapple chunks, fresh or canned in juice (not syrup) and drained.

Nutrition Facts
Each serving about:

Calories	481	Total fat	13 g	Vitamin C	63 mg
Protein	44 g	Saturated fat	1 g	Calcium	241 mg
Carbohydrate	52 g	Cholesterol	73 mg	Fiber	11 g
		Sodium	747 mg	Omega-3	390 mg

SNACKS (about 125 calories each)

Blueberry Lassi

Blend ¼ cup frozen blueberries or mango cubes with ½ cup each plain fat-free yogurt and fat-free (skim) milk; if desired, add zero-calorie sweetener to taste.

Each serving about: 121 calories, 10 g protein, 19 g carbohydrate, 0 g total fat (0 g saturated fat), 5 mg cholesterol, 142 mg sodium, 2 mg vitamin C, 381 mg calcium, 1 g fiber, 40 mg omega-3

Cantaloupe Boat

Mix ⅓ cup plain fat-free Greek yogurt with zero-calorie sweetener to taste; serve in the center of ½ fresh small (4¼-inch) cantaloupe; if desired, garnish with fresh mint leaves.

Each serving about: 115 calories, 9 g protein, 21 g carbohydrate, 0 g total fat (0 g saturated fat), 0 mg cholesterol, 64 mg sodium, 81 mg vitamin C, 109 mg calcium, 2 g fiber, 100 mg omega-3

Cheese Bite

1 Mini Babybel Sharp Original or Gouda with 1 can (5½ ounces) low-sodium or spicy hot vegetable juice.

Each serving about: 113 calories, 6 g protein, 6 g carbohydrate, 6 g total fat (4 g saturated fat), 20 mg cholesterol, 260 mg sodium, 46 mg vitamin C, 112 mg calcium, 1 g fiber, 0 mg omega-3

Cherries & Cheese

1 (¾-ounce) wedge aged goat cheese or Brie served with 10 cherries or 2 tablespoons dried tart cherries.

Each serving about: 109 calories, 5 g protein, 13 g carbohydrate, 5 g total fat (3 g saturated fat), 10 mg cholesterol, 78 mg sodium, 6 mg vitamin C, 40 mg calcium, 2 g fiber, 20 mg omega-3

Chips & Cheese

5 Food Should Taste Good Multigrain Chips with 1 mozzarella stick.

Each serving about: 131 calories, 8 g protein, 11 g carbohydrate, 3 g total fat (2 g saturated fat), 10 mg cholesterol, 226 mg sodium, 0 mg vitamin C, 165 mg calcium, 2 g fiber, 0 mg omega-3

Citrus Snack

½ pink grapefruit sprinkled with zero-calorie sweetener to taste; serve with ½ cup 1% low-sodium cottage cheese.

Each serving about: 127 calories, 15 g protein, 15 g carbohydrate, 1 g total fat (1 g saturated fat), 5 mg cholesterol, 16 mg sodium, 47 mg vitamin C, 82 mg calcium, 2 g fiber, 20 mg omega-3

Cocoa Fix

12 Emerald Cocoa Roast Almonds (dark-chocolate flavor) or other flavored almonds and ½ cup fat-free (skim) milk.

Each serving about: 124 calories, 7 g protein, 9 g carbohydrate, 7 g total fat (1 g saturated fat), 2 mg cholesterol, 52 mg sodium, 0 mg vitamin C, 191 mg calcium, 2 g fiber, 0 mg omega-3

Edamame Munchie

¼ cup Seapoint Farms Dry Roasted Edamame, lightly salted or wasabi flavor.

Each serving about: 130 calories, 14 g protein, 10 g carbohydrate, 4 g total fat (1 g saturated fat), 0 mg cholesterol, 150 mg sodium, 1 mg vitamin C, 40 mg calcium, 8 g fiber, 0 mg omega-3

Fruit & Grain Bar

1 Kashi Chewy Cherry Dark Chocolate Granola Bar.

Each serving about: *120 calories, 5 g protein, 24 g carbohydrate, 2 g total fat (1 g saturated fat), 0 mg cholesterol, 65 mg sodium, 0 mg vitamin C, 0 mg calcium, 4 g fiber, 0 mg omega-3*

Honeydew "Sundae"

Top 1⅓ cups honeydew melon chunks with ⅓ cup plain fat-free Greek yogurt; sprinkle with 2 teaspoons fresh mint leaves.

Each serving about: *122 calories, 8 g protein, 24 g carbohydrate, 0 g total fat (0 g saturated fat), 0 mg cholesterol, 70 mg sodium, 41 mg vitamin C, 104 mg calcium, 2 g fiber, 70 mg omega-3*

Hummus & Veggie Strips

¼ cup hummus with ½ large red bell pepper, cut into strips (about ¾ cup).

Each serving about: *125 calories, 6 g protein, 13 g carbohydrate, 6 g total fat (1 g saturated fat), 0 mg cholesterol, 240 mg sodium, 88 mg vitamin C, 29 mg calcium, 5 g fiber, 20 mg omega-3*

Iced-Coffee Break

1 (16-ounce) nonfat iced sugar-free flavored latte with 1 piece Dove Dark Chocolate Promises.

Each serving about: *120 calories, 8 g protein, 17 g carbohydrate, 3 g total fat (2 g saturated fat), 6 mg cholesterol, 0 mg sodium, 0 mg vitamin C, 150 mg calcium, 1 g fiber, 0 mg omega-3*

Movie Mix

Combine 1 cup Good Health Half Naked Popcorn or air-popped popcorn with 1½ tablespoons dried-plum bits or raisins and 15 shelled roasted unsalted pistachios.

Each serving about: *131 calories, 3 g protein, 20 g carbohydrate, 5 g total fat (1 g saturated fat), 0 mg cholesterol, 5 mg sodium, 0 mg vitamin C, 18 mg calcium, 3 g fiber, 20 mg omega-3*

Out & About

1 Kind Mini Fruit & Nut Delight Bar with 5 grapes.

Each serving about: *116 calories, 3 g protein, 14 g carbohydrate, 6 g total fat (1 g saturated fat), 0 mg cholesterol, 10 mg sodium, 2 mg vitamin C, 22 mg calcium, 2 g fiber, 0 mg omega-3*

PB & J–Inspired Yogurt

¾ cup fat-free Greek yogurt topped with 1 teaspoon each no-sugar-added grape jam and chopped unsalted roasted peanuts.

Each serving about: *116 calories, 16 g protein, 10 g carbohydrate, 2 g total fat (0 g saturated fat), 0 mg cholesterol, 65 mg sodium, 0 mg vitamin C, 202 mg calcium, 0 g fiber, 0 mg omega-3*

Pineapple Plate

Arrange ½ cup fresh or grilled pineapple cubes on a bed of ½ cup 1% low-sodium cottage cheese; sprinkle with 2 teaspoons pomegranate seeds.

Each serving about: *128 calories, 15 g protein, 15 g carbohydrate, 1 g total fat (1 g saturated fat), 5 mg cholesterol, 15 mg sodium, 40 mg vitamin C, 80 mg calcium, 1 g fiber, 20 mg omega-3*

Pistachios

Have 30 pistachios.

Each serving about: 118 calories, 4 g protein, 6 g carbohydrate, 9 g total fat (1 g saturated fat), 0 mg cholesterol, 0 mg sodium, 1 mg vitamin C, 23 mg calcium, 2 g fiber, 50 mg omega-3

Prosciutto & Mozzarella Plate

Arrange ½ ounce very thinly sliced prosciutto and 1 ounce thinly sliced part-skim mozzarella on a plate; top with ¼ cup cantaloupe cubes and drizzle with ½ teaspoon balsamic vinegar.

Each serving about: 118 calories, 11 g protein, 5 g carbohydrate, 6 g total fat (3 g saturated fat), 29 mg cholesterol, 562 mg sodium, 15 mg vitamin C, 226 mg calcium, 0 g fiber, 60 mg omega-3

Pudding Parfait

Stir ½ teaspoon grated lemon peel into 1 single-serve container sugar-free vanilla pudding and layer in a beverage glass with 1 cup blackberries or blueberries.

Each serving about: 122 calories, 2 g protein, 25 g carbohydrate, 4 g total fat (2 g saturated fat), 0 mg cholesterol, 102 mg sodium, 32 mg vitamin C, 143 mg calcium, 7 g fiber, 140 mg omega-3

Ricotta-Fig Toasts

Cut a 1-ounce piece of whole-grain fruit-nut bread in half diagonally. Toast, if desired, and top each half with 1 tablespoon part-skim ricotta cheese, ½ teaspoon honey, and ½ dried fig.

Each serving about: 119 calories, 5 g protein, 22 g carbohydrate, 2 g total fat (1 g saturated fat), 6 mg cholesterol, 26 mg sodium, 0 mg vitamin C, 49 mg calcium, 4 g fiber, 0 mg omega-3

Strawberry Bagel Thin

Spread ½ of a toasted 100% Whole Wheat Thomas' Bagel Thin with 1 wedge Laughing Cow ⅓ Less Fat Classic Cream Cheese Spread. Slice 3 large strawberries, toss with ½ teaspoon fresh lemon juice, and arrange atop cheese spread.

Each serving about: 118 calories, 5 g protein, 16 g carbohydrate, 5 g total fat (3 g saturated fat), 10 mg cholesterol, 236 mg sodium, 33 mg vitamin C, 129 mg calcium, 4 g fiber, 40 mg omega-3

Strawberry Sipper

1 cup fat-free milk blended with ¾ cup frozen sliced strawberries and ½ teaspoon pure vanilla extract.

Each serving about: 124 calories, 9 g protein, 22 g carbohydrate, 0 g total fat (0 g saturated fat), 5 mg cholesterol, 105 mg sodium, 46 mg vitamin C, 324 mg calcium, 2 g fiber, 30 mg omega-3

Veggies & Dill Dip

Combine 3 tablespoons plain fat-free Greek yogurt, 1 tablespoon light mayonnaise, and a dash each of fresh or dried dill and garlic salt; serve with 1 medium zucchini, sliced, and 8 cherry tomatoes.

Each serving about: 122 calories, 8 g protein, 12 g carbohydrate, 6 g total fat (1 g saturated fat), 5 mg cholesterol, 243 mg sodium, 56 mg vitamin C, 93 mg calcium, 3 g fiber, 120 mg omega-3

Yogurt Sundae

1 container Chobani Bites Raspberry with Dark Chocolate Chips flavor, served with 5 raspberries and 5 pistachios.

Each serving about: 122 calories, 9 g protein, 15 g carbohydrate, 1 g total fat (0 g saturated fat), 0 mg cholesterol, 960 mg sodium, 3 mg vitamin C, 106 mg calcium, 1 g fiber, 20 mg omega-3

7 Quick & Easy Dinners...

From a Rotisserie Chicken

When just the thought of cooking dinner overwhelms you, pick up a precooked rotisserie chicken. They're available from most markets or your local chicken takeout. Each satisfying serving of these recipes is 515 calories or less, provided you toss the skin. And because they require only five ingredients (not including the chicken, oil, salt, and pepper) and a minimum of chopping, you can have these meals ready in 25 minutes or less—and keep your can-do spirit high.

Arugula & Cranberry Salad

In large bowl, toss 1 package (5 ounces) baby arugula, ¼ cup dried cranberries, 3 tablespoons light balsamic vinaigrette, and ¼ teaspoon freshly ground black pepper. Divide among 4 plates. Top with sliced meat from 1 rotisserie chicken. With vegetable peeler, shave 1 ounce Parmesan cheese over all. Serve with whole-grain dinner rolls. Serves 4.

Each serving about: 461 calories, 49 g protein, 27 g carbohydrate, 19 g total fat (7 g saturated fat), 157 mg cholesterol, 1,291 mg sodium, 6 mg vitamin C, 388 mg calcium, 3 g fiber, 90 mg omega-3

BBQ Chicken Slaw

In large bowl, toss 1 bag (14 ounces) coleslaw mix; shredded meat from 1 rotisserie chicken; 1 can (15¼ ounces) no-salt-added corn kernels, rinsed and drained; ⅓ cup barbecue sauce; and 1 tablespoon cider vinegar. Serve with or on whole wheat hamburger buns. Serves 4.

Each serving about: 502 calories, 44 g protein, 56 g carbohydrate, 12 g total fat (3 g saturated fat), 137 mg cholesterol, 1,111 mg sodium, 32 mg vitamin C, 97 mg calcium, 9 g fiber, 50 mg omega-3

Black Bean Burritos

In large bowl, toss half 10-ounce bag chopped romaine lettuce; shredded meat from 1 rotisserie chicken; 1 can (14½ ounces) no-salt-added black beans, rinsed and drained; and 1 cup fresh salsa. Warm 4 large whole wheat tortillas as label directs. Divide chicken mixture among tortillas and wrap. Serves 4.

Each serving about: 500 calories, 46 g protein, 45 g carbohydrate, 13 g total fat (3 g saturated fat), 137 mg cholesterol, 1,146 mg sodium, 44 mg vitamin C, 144 mg calcium, 7 g fiber, 0 mg omega-3

Cheesy Chicken Casserole

Preheat oven to 425°F. In 8" by 8" baking dish, stir together 1 pound frozen cut green beans, thawed; ½ cup marinara sauce; and 2 tablespoons sliced pimientos, drained, until combined. Top with shredded meat from 1 rotisserie chicken and ½ cup marinara sauce. Sprinkle with 1 cup shredded part-skim mozzarella cheese. Bake 15 minutes or until cheese melts. Serve with multigrain dinner rolls. Serves 4.

Each serving about: 504 calories, 49 g protein, 34 g carbohydrate, 19 g total fat (7 g saturated fat), 154 mg cholesterol, 1,166 mg sodium, 13 mg vitamin C, 307 mg calcium, 7 g fiber, 100 mg omega-3

Soba Salad

Heat 4-quart saucepan of water to boiling on high. Cook 12 ounces soba noodles as label directs. Drain; rinse with cold water. Drain well. Transfer to large bowl along with 3 cups mixed greens, 3 ounces shredded skinless chicken breast, 2 cups shredded carrots, 4 tablespoons dry-roasted peanuts, ⅓ cup light ginger salad dressing, and ⅛ teaspoon freshly ground black pepper. Toss until well coated. Serves 4.

Each serving about: 496 calories, 36 g protein, 77 g carbohydrate, 9 g total fat (1 g saturated fat), 52 mg cholesterol, 1,274 mg sodium, 3 mg vitamin C, 55 mg calcium, 3 g fiber, 10 mg omega-3

Spinach & Beet Salad

In large bowl, toss 1 package (5 ounces) baby spinach; 1 package (8 ounces) precooked peeled baby beets, cut into quarters; 3 tablespoons light poppy seed dressing; and ⅛ teaspoon freshly ground black pepper. Divide among 4 plates. Top with sliced meat from 1 rotisserie chicken; 8 tablespoons dry-roasted, salted soy nuts; and 1 tablespoon dressing. Serve with whole-grain rolls. Serves 4.

Each serving about: 473 calories, 45 g protein, 38 g carbohydrate, 17 g total fat (4 g saturated fat), 142 mg cholesterol, 1,056 mg sodium, 7 mg vitamin C, 79 mg calcium, 5 g fiber, 30 mg omega-3

Stuffed Pitas

In large bowl, whisk together ½ cup roasted red pepper hummus, 2 tablespoons lemon juice, 1 tablespoon water, and ⅛ teaspoon freshly ground black pepper. Add 2 cups shredded meat from 1 rotisserie chicken and 5 cups Italian-blend mixed greens; toss until combined. Divide mixture among 4 whole wheat pita pockets, toasted. Serves 4.

Each serving about: 480 calories, 45 g protein, 46 carbohydrate, 15 g total fat (3 g saturated fat), 137 mg cholesterol, 1,145 mg sodium, 5 mg vitamin C, 10 mg calcium, 7 g fiber, 30 mg omega-3

7 Quick & Easy Dinners...

From Whole Wheat Pasta

Each of the weeknight-friendly recipes below calls for 12 ounces of uncooked whole wheat pasta and up to five from-the-pantry and already-prepared ingredients, not including salt or pepper. With a minimum of chopping, you'll have a healthy dinner—with no more than 538 calories per serving and plenty of fill-you-up fiber, and low in saturated fat—on the table in 30 minutes or less. If you have a whole wheat pasta of a similar shape in your cabinet, feel free to swap it in.

Creamy Peas & Ham Pasta

Cook penne as label directs; reserve ½ cup pasta water. Drain pasta; return to pot. Stir in 10 ounces frozen peas, thawed; 2 cups baby spinach; 1 cup part-skim ricotta cheese; 4 ounces thinly sliced low-sodium deli ham; reserved pasta cooking water; and ¼ teaspoon each salt and freshly ground black pepper. Serves 4.

Each serving about: 494 calories, 27 g protein, 79 g carbohydrate, 8 g total fat (3 g saturated fat), 34 mg cholesterol, 557 mg sodium, 15 mg vitamin C, 224 mg calcium, 11 g fiber, 60 mg omega-3

Fall Sausage & Veggie Pasta

Heat 1 tablespoon olive oil in 12-inch skillet on medium-high. Add 1 package (20 ounces) peeled and cut butternut squash; 2 links low-fat precooked chicken sausage, sliced; and 4 cloves garlic, crushed with press. Cook 4 minutes or until browned, stirring occasionally. Reduce heat to medium. Add 1 cup water, cover, and cook 8 minutes or until squash is tender. Cook spaghetti as label directs; reserve ½ cup pasta water. Drain and add to squash mixture along with 1 package (10 ounces) frozen chopped spinach, thawed; reserved pasta cooking water; and ¼ teaspoon freshly ground black pepper. Toss until well mixed. Serves 4.

Each serving about: 505 calories, 23 g protein, 85 g carbohydrate, 11 g total fat (2 g saturated fat), 40 mg cholesterol, 480 mg sodium, 32 mg vitamin C, 176 mg calcium, 15 g fiber, 90 mg omega-3

Italian Tuna Pasta

Cook penne as label directs. Meanwhile, in 3-quart saucepan, heat 1 tablespoon olive oil on medium-high; add 8 ounces sliced cremini mushrooms and cook on medium 7 minutes or until mushrooms have softened, stirring occasionally. Stir in 2 cans (5 ounces each) chunk light tuna in water, drained; 1 cup marinara sauce; 2 tablespoons capers, rinsed and drained; and 1/8 teaspoon freshly ground black pepper; heat through. Reserve 1/2 cup pasta water. Drain pasta; return to pot along with tuna mixture and reserved pasta cooking water. Stir until well coated. Serves 4.

Each serving about: 538 calories, 32 g protein, 75 g carbohydrate, 11 g total fat (1 g saturated fat), 45 mg cholesterol, 696 mg sodium, 1 mg vitamin C, 57 mg calcium, 10 g fiber, 80 mg omega-3

Mac & Cheese Pasta

In 5-quart saucepan, whisk 2 1/2 cups low-fat (1%) milk into 2 tablespoons cornstarch. Heat to boiling on medium, whisking, and cook 2 minutes to thicken. Reduce heat to low; stir in 5 ounces shredded reduced-fat (50%) Cheddar cheese until melted. Meanwhile, cook penne 2 minutes less than label directs. To pasta in pot, add 1 package (1 pound) frozen broccoli-cauliflower mix; cook 2 minutes. Drain; stir into cheese mixture along with 1/4 teaspoon freshly ground black pepper. Serves 4.

Each serving about: 533 calories, 26 g protein, 82 g carbohydrate, 11 g total fat (5 g saturated fat), 33 mg cholesterol, 407 mg sodium, 36 mg vitamin C, 745 mg calcium, 10 g fiber, 10 mg omega-3

Mediterranean Feta & Tomato Pasta

Cook spaghetti 2 minutes less than label directs. To pasta in pot, add 1 can (14 1/2 ounces) lower-sodium white (cannellini) beans, rinsed and drained, and 1 pint grape tomatoes; cook 2 minutes. Reserve 1/4 cup pasta water; drain and immediately transfer to large bowl. Toss with 9 cups (5-ounce bag) baby arugula, 3/4 cup crumbled feta cheese, reserved pasta cooking water, and 1/4 teaspoon freshly ground black pepper. Serves 4.

Each serving about: 472 calories, 23 g protein, 83 g carbohydrate, 8 g total fat (4 g saturated fat), 25 mg cholesterol, 366 mg sodium, 15 mg vitamin C, 268 mg calcium, 16 g fiber, 150 mg omega-3

Spring Shrimp Pasta

From 1 lemon, grate 1 tablespoon peel and squeeze 2 tablespoons juice. Cook spaghetti 4 minutes less than label directs. To pasta in pot, add 2 pounds asparagus, trimmed and cut into 2-inch lengths, and 12 ounces shelled, deveined shrimp; cook 4 minutes or until pasta is cooked. Reserve 1/4 cup pasta water. Drain pasta; return to pot. Stir in 2 tablespoons extra virgin olive oil, reserved lemon peel and juice, reserved pasta cooking water, and 1/4 teaspoon each salt and freshly ground black pepper. Serves 4.

Each serving about: 529 calories, 35 g protein, 74 g carbohydrate, 13 g total fat (2 g saturated fat), 129 mg cholesterol, 283 mg sodium, 20 mg vitamin C, 136 mg calcium, 16 g fiber, 530 mg omega-3

Tofu Lo Mein

Cook spaghetti 1 minute less than label directs. To pasta in pot, add 1 package (14 ounces) coleslaw mix and 1 package (8 ounces) stringless snap peas; cook 1 minute. Drain and immediately transfer to large bowl. Toss with 1 box (14 ounces) firm tofu, drained and cut up; ⅓ cup lower-sodium teriyaki sauce; 1 tablespoon toasted sesame oil; and ¼ teaspoon freshly ground black pepper. Serves 4.

Each serving about: *475 calories, 24 g protein, 79 g carbohydrate, 10 g total fat (1 g saturated fat), 0 mg cholesterol, 379 mg sodium, 63 mg vitamin C, 296 mg calcium, 15 g fiber, 20 mg omega-3*

7 Quick & Easy Dinners...

From Canned Beans

If you're looking for the fountain of youth, you might find it in a can of beans. Beans are rich in fiber, including the soluble kind that helps reduce dangerous belly fat. Reducing your meat consumption by bulking up recipes with beans has many advantages. It's a strategy that may help lower your risk of age-related illnesses like heart disease and cancer. And since beans run less than $2 per can, they're an inexpensive way to boost protein in recipes. Just one bean bummer: Like many convenience foods, canned beans are high in sodium—not a worry on the 7 Years Younger Meal Plan, since most of our meals keep the salt in check. Also, rinsing the beans, as we do in the recipes below, slashes about a third of their sodium. Thanks to the use of pre-chopped and -shredded veggies, these easy dinners can be prepped in 30 minutes max—less time than it can take to get a pizza delivered!

Bangers & White Bean Mash

Preheat grill on medium-high. Grill 8 links spicy Italian turkey sausage 8 minutes or until cooked through, turning occasionally; transfer to cutting board and cover with foil. Meanwhile, in 3-quart saucepot, heat 1½ (15-ounce) cans lower-sodium cannellini beans, rinsed and drained; 3 cloves garlic, crushed with press; ½ cup nonfat milk; and 2 teaspoons extra virgin olive oil on medium-high and cook 5 minutes, mashing with potato masher until mostly smooth. Serve sausages with white bean mash and 6 cups baby spinach, wilted. Serves 4.

Each serving about: 500 calories, 51 g protein, 25 g carbohydrate, 22 g total fat (4 g saturated fat), 157 mg cholesterol, 1,375 mg sodium, 15 mg vitamin C, 171 mg calcium, 7 g fiber, 370 mg omega-3

Chicken & Garbanzo Bean Piccata

Cook 1¼ cups bulgur as label directs. Meanwhile, in 12-inch skillet, heat 2 tablespoons extra virgin olive oil on medium-high. Sprinkle 1¼ pounds thin chicken-breast cutlets with ⅛ teaspoon salt. Add chicken to skillet; cook 5 minutes or until browned, turning over once. Transfer to plate. To skillet, add 3 tablespoons lemon juice; 2 cloves garlic, crushed with press; and 2 tablespoons capers, chopped. Cook 1 minute. Add 10 ounces fresh spinach and ¼ teaspoon salt. Cook 1 minute, stirring. Return chicken to skillet along with 1 (15-ounce) can lower-sodium garbanzo beans, rinsed and drained. Cook 2 minutes or until chicken is cooked through (165°F). Serve chicken, beans, and spinach over bulgur. Serves 4.

Each serving about: 505 calories, 44 g protein, 56 g carbohydrate, 12 g total fat (2 g saturated fat), 14 g fiber, 91 mg cholesterol, 600 mg sodium, 27 mg vitamin C, 139 mg calcium, 14 g fiber, 200 mg omega-3

Grilled Chicken Salad

Preheat grill or grill pan on medium-high. In medium bowl, toss 8 ounces chicken tenders with 1 tablespoon canola oil; sprinkle with ½ teaspoon ground coriander and ⅛ teaspoon salt. Grill chicken 5 to 7 minutes or until cooked through (165°F), turning over once. Slice each chicken tender and add to bowl, along with 4 cups arugula; 2 (15-ounce) cans lower-sodium garbanzo beans, rinsed and drained; ½ cup bottled red wine vinaigrette; and 1 English (seedless) cucumber, sliced. Toss to combine. Serve with 3 small (4-inch) whole wheat pitas, cut into quarters and toasted. Serves 4.

Each serving about: 485 calories, 26 g protein, 55 g carbohydrate, 17 g total fat (3 g saturated fat), 31 mg cholesterol, 700 mg sodium, 7 mg vitamin C, 126 mg calcium, 11 g fiber, 90 mg omega-3

Light Shrimp & White Bean Scampi

In 12-inch skillet, heat 2 tablespoons extra virgin olive oil on medium-high. Add 1 pound frozen shelled, deveined shrimp, thawed; 1 (15-ounce) can lower-sodium cannellini beans, rinsed and drained; 3 Tbsp. lemon juice; 2 cloves garlic, crushed with press; and ¼ teaspoon salt; cook 3 to 5 minutes or until shrimp are cooked through, stirring occasionally. Stir in 10 ounces baby spinach and cook 2 minutes or until wilted. Stir in ½ cup chopped parsley. Serve shrimp mixture over 2 (10-ounce) bags frozen brown rice, cooked. Serves 4.

Each serving about: 505 calories, 27 g protein, 64 g carbohydrate, 12 g total fat (1 g saturated fat), 143 mg cholesterol, 950 mg sodium, 25 mg vitamin C, 157 mg calcium, 10 g fiber, 130 mg omega-3

Spaghetti with Green Olive Pesto

In large pot of boiling salted water, cook 12 ounces whole-grain spaghetti as label directs; drain pasta, reserving ½ cup pasta water, and transfer to large bowl. Meanwhile, in food processor, pulse ¾ cup pitted green olives, ½ cup each packed parsley and basil leaves, and 2 tablespoons extra virgin olive oil until mixture is coarsely ground. Add pesto to bowl with spaghetti along with 1 (15-ounce) can lower-sodium cannellini beans, rinsed and drained; ½ teaspoon crushed red pepper; ¼ cup grated Parmesan cheese; and ¼ to ½ cup reserved pasta cooking water. Serves 4.

Each serving about: 500 calories, 20 g protein, 80 g carbohydrate, 14 g total fat (3 g saturated fat), 4 mg cholesterol, 585 mg sodium, 11 mg vitamin C, 153 mg calcium, 15 g fiber, 120 mg omega-3

Vegetarian Spicy Bean Burgers

In large bowl, with potato masher, mash 2 (15-ounce) cans lower-sodium pinto beans, rinsed and drained; 1 tablespoon hot pepper sauce; 1 clove garlic, crushed with press; ½ teaspoon ground cumin; and ¼ teaspoon salt until almost smooth. Stir in ¾ cup whole wheat bread crumbs; firmly press into 4 (1-inch-thick) patties. In 12-inch nonstick skillet, heat 3 tablespoons canola oil on medium 1 minute. Cook patties 10 minutes or until golden brown, turning over once. Serve on 4 whole wheat hamburger buns. Divide 1 avocado, sliced, and ½ cup salsa among burgers.

Each serving about: 490 calories, 16 g protein, 68 g carbohydrate, 19 g total fat (2 g saturated fat), 0 mg cholesterol, 900 mg sodium, 7 mg vitamin C, 140 mg calcium, 19 g fiber, 1,080 mg omega-3

Veggie Casserole

Heat oven to 400°F. In large bowl, combine 2 (15-ounce) cans lower-sodium black beans, rinsed and drained; 2 cups frozen corn, thawed; 1 cup shredded carrots; 1 cup canned tomato sauce; ½ cup crumbled feta; 2 cloves garlic, crushed with press; and ½ teaspoon chili powder. In 2-quart baking dish, layer 1 cup coarsely crushed baked whole-grain tortilla chips, then vegetable mixture. Top with 1 cup coarsely crushed baked whole-grain tortilla chips. Bake 15 minutes or until heated through. Serves 4.

Each serving about: 480 calories, 22 g protein, 79 g carbohydrate, 10 g total fat (4 g saturated fat), 18 mg cholesterol, 960 mg sodium, 11 mg vitamin C, 232 mg calcium, 15 g fiber, 70 mg omega-3

7 Quick & Easy Dinners...

From Canned Tuna

Our panelists asked for speedy meals, and we listened! Each of the recipes below can be ready to eat in 30 minutes or less, thanks to shortcuts like jarred salsa, frozen vegetables, and bottled salad dressings. Starring always-in-the-pantry canned tuna, they're also wallet-friendly. At 30 cents per ounce, canned light tuna is one of the most inexpensive sources of youth-boosting omega-3s you can find. For about 15 cents more per ounce, canned white (albacore) tuna packs about three times as much of these inflammation-fighting fish fats. However, this variety also has more mercury. For most healthy people, the benefits outweigh the risks, but if you're pregnant or breastfeeding, or if you're feeding children, have no more than 6 ounces of white tuna per week (about two of these recipes).

Dill Tuna Burgers

Mix 2 (5-ounce) cans tuna, drained; 4 green onions, chopped; 2 stalks celery, chopped; ¾ cup whole wheat bread crumbs; ¼ cup tartar sauce; ¼ cup chopped fresh dill; 1 tablespoon lemon juice; 1 teaspoon hot pepper sauce; ½ teaspoon salt; and ¼ teaspoon pepper to combine. In 12-inch nonstick skillet, heat 1 tablespoon extra virgin olive oil on medium-high. Firmly press tuna mixture into 4 patties; add to skillet and cook 3 minutes per side or until heated through. Divide tuna burgers, 4 leaves Bibb lettuce, ¼ cup tartar sauce, and 2 ounces reduced-fat potato chips (about 36 chips) among 4 toasted whole-grain buns. Serves 4.

Each serving about: *470 calories, 20 g protein, 45 g carbohydrate, 23 g total fat (3 g saturated fat), 29 mg cholesterol, 1,060 mg sodium, 14 mg vitamin C, 91 mg calcium, 6 g fiber, 660 mg omega-3*

Smoky Tuna Pasta

In 5-quart saucepot, heat 2 tablespoons extra virgin olive oil on medium-high. Add 1 large red pepper, sliced; 2 cups shredded carrots; 2 tablespoons water; and ¼ teaspoon salt. Cover; cook 8 minutes or until tender, stirring occasionally. Add ¾ cup frozen peas, thawed; 2 cups marinara sauce; 2 (5-ounce) cans tuna, drained; and 1 teaspoon smoked paprika. Cook 2 minutes, stirring. Toss with 8 ounces whole wheat spaghetti, cooked, and 2 tablespoons grated Parmesan cheese. Serves 4.

Each serving about: 510 calories, 27 g protein, 72 g carbohydrate, 14 g total fat (3 g saturated fat), 29 mg cholesterol, 965 mg sodium, 60 mg vitamin C, 109 mg calcium, 14 g fiber, 690 mg omega-3

Tuna & Bulgur Lettuce Cups

Cook 1¼ cups bulgur as label directs; cool slightly. Meanwhile, in large microwave-safe bowl, combine 12 ounces trimmed green beans, sliced, and 1 tablespoon water. Cover with vented plastic wrap; microwave on High 5 minutes or until tender. Drain; add 1 cup bottled light sesame vinaigrette along with 2 (5-ounce) cans tuna, drained, stirring to combine. Serve bulgur in butter lettuce leaves topped with tuna mixture and ½ cup roasted, salted peanuts, chopped. Serves 4.

Each serving about: 485 calories, 27 g protein, 58 g carbohydrate, 18 g total fat (1 g saturated fat), 24 mg cholesterol, 880 mg sodium, 10 mg vitamin C, 94 mg calcium, 12 g fiber, 700 mg omega-3

Tuna & Zucchini Tacos

Preheat grill or large grill pan on medium-high. Toss 2 medium zucchini, sliced, with 1 tablespoon canola oil, ½ teaspoon chili powder, and ⅛ teaspoon salt; grill 5 minutes, turning over once. Transfer zucchini to large bowl along with 2 (5-ounce) cans tuna, drained, and 2 cups frozen corn, thawed. In medium bowl, stir together ½ cup chunky salsa and ¼ teaspoon chipotle chile powder. Serve tuna mixture with salsa, fresh cilantro leaves, 1 cup prepared guacamole, and 8 whole wheat soft taco-size tortillas. Serves 4.

Each serving about: 480 calories, 27 g protein, 67 g carbohydrate, 15 g total fat (6 g saturated fat), 34 mg cholesterol, 1,395 mg sodium, 27 mg vitamin C, 30 mg calcium, 9 g fiber, 640 mg omega-3

Tuna Melts

In medium bowl, mix 2 (5-ounce) cans tuna, drained; ½ cup chopped celery; ¼ cup mayonnaise; 1 teaspoon each red wine vinegar and Dijon mustard; and ½ teaspoon crushed red pepper. Top 4 slices bread with tuna mixture, 1 sliced avocado, 1 slice each American cheese, and 2 slices each reduced-sodium dill pickle. Top with 4 slices bread; transfer to foil-lined cookie sheet and broil 2 minutes or until cheese melts. Serves 4.

Each serving about: 470 calories, 27 g protein, 29 g carbohydrate, 26 g total fat (7 g saturated fat), 49 mg cholesterol, 945 mg sodium, 4 mg vitamin C, 277 mg calcium, 7 g fiber, 730 mg omega-3

Tuna Niçoise Tartine

Cook 1 (12-ounce) bag microwavable green beans as label directs; transfer to large bowl, add 2 tablespoons bottled balsamic vinaigrette, and toss to combine. Toss 2 (5-ounce) cans tuna, drained, with 4 tablespoons bottled balsamic vinaigrette. Split 1 loaf whole-grain baguette in half lengthwise, then cut in half again to make 4 pieces; toast and top with 1 large tomato, sliced; green beans with dressing; tuna; 2/3 cup pitted Niçoise olives; 8 sliced hard-cooked eggs; and 1/2 cup packed basil leaves. Serves 4.

Each serving about: 490 calories, 33 g protein, 35 g carbohydrate, 24 g total fat (5 g saturated fat), 397 mg cholesterol, 910 mg sodium, 18 mg vitamin C, 120 mg calcium, 6 g fiber, 720 mg omega-3

"Unfried" Rice

In 12-inch nonstick skillet, heat 2 tablespoons sesame oil on medium. Add 2 cups shredded carrots; 1 1/2 cups frozen peas, thawed; 2 tablespoons water; and 1/8 teaspoon salt. Cook 5 minutes or until tender, stirring occasionally. Add 4 cups cooked brown rice, 3 large eggs, and 1 bunch green onions, sliced. Cook 2 minutes, stirring. Add 2 (5-ounce) cans tuna, drained; 2 tablespoons soy sauce; and 1 tablespoon unseasoned rice vinegar. Cook 1 minute or until heated through, stirring. Serves 4.

Each serving about: 480 calories, 28 g protein, 61 g carbohydrate, 14 g total fat (3 g saturated fat), 163 mg cholesterol, 845 mg sodium, 13 mg vitamin C, 93 mg calcium, 8 g fiber, 660 mg omega-3

BREAD SWAPS

Consider this Carb Lover Central. The chart below shows you how to customize your sandwich, wrap, roll—even your waffle—by swapping it out for another bread item. Let the calories steer you to an equivalent item. And don't forget to take a close look at the portion size. We listed the manufacturers' serving information—in some cases, three slices of bread—so adjust accordingly.

Brand	Whole-Grain Option	Calories	Serving Size
La Tortilla Factory	Smart & Delicious White Whole Wheat Soft Wraps Mini	50	1 wrap
La Tortilla Factory	Smart & Delicious Multibran Soft Wraps Mini	50	1 wrap
La Tortilla Factory	Smart & Delicious Three Seed Soft Wraps Mini	50	1 wrap
Nature's Own	100% Whole Wheat (20-oz. loaf)	50	1 slice
Nature's Own	100% Whole Grain Sugar Free Bread	50	1 slice
Nature's Own	Double Fiber Wheat Bread	50	1 slice
Nature's Own	100% Whole Grain Bread	70	1 slice
Pepperidge Farm	Whole Grain Rye Bread	70	1 slice
Generic (no brand)	Whole Wheat Dinner Rolls (1 to 1½ oz.)	75-115	1 roll
Arnold	100% Whole Wheat Bakery Light	80	2 slices
Food for Life	Ezekiel 4:9 Sprouted 100% Whole Grain Cinnamon Raisin Bread	80	1 slice
Food for Life	Ezekiel 4:9 Low Sodium Whole Grain Bread	80	1 slice
Food for Life	Ezekiel 4:9 Flax Sprouted Whole Grain Bread	80	1 slice
Food for Life	Ezekiel 4:9 Sesame Sprouted Whole Grain Bread	80	1 slice
Food for Life	Ezekiel 4:9 Sprouted Whole Grain Bread	80	1 slice
Food for Life	Ezekiel 4:9 Taco Size Whole Grain Tortillas	80	1 tortilla

Brand	Whole-Grain Option	Calories	Serving Size
Nature's Own	40 Calorie 9 Grain Bread	80	2 slices
Food for Life	7 Whole Grain Pocket Bread	90	1 pocket bread
Sara Lee	Hearty & Delicious Healthy Multi-Grain Bread	90	1 slice
Arnold/Brownberry	100% Whole Wheat Pocket Thins	100	½ slice pocket thin
Arnold/Brown-berry/Oroweat	100% Whole Wheat Pocket or Sandwich Thins	100	1 roll
Flatout	Soft 100% Whole Wheat Flatbread	100	1 flatbread
Flatout	Multi-Grain with Flax Flatbread	100	1 flatbread
Food for Life	Ezekiel Whole Grain Pocket Bread	100	1 pocket bread
La Tortilla Factory	100 Calorie Whole Wheat Tortillas	100	1 tortilla
La Tortilla Factory	Extra Virgin Olive Oil Soft Wraps in Multigrain	100	1 wrap
La Tortilla Factory	Extra Virgin Olive Oil Soft Wraps in Whole Grain White	100	1 wrap
Mission	Artisan Style Tortillas in Multigrain	100	1 tortilla
Nature's Own	100% Whole Wheat Sandwich Rounds	100	1 round
Nature's Own	100% Whole Grain Sandwich Rounds	100	1 round
Nature's Own	100% Whole Wheat Hot Dog Rolls	100	1 roll
Pepperidge Farm	Whole Grain 100% Whole Wheat Bread	100	1 slice
Pepperidge Farm	100% Natural German Dark Wheat Bread	100	1 slice
Pepperidge Farm	100% Whole Wheat Bagel Flats	100	1 bagel flat
Pepperidge Farm	Deli Flats Soft 100% Whole Wheat Thin Rolls	100	1 roll
Mission	Multigrain Small/Fajita Flour Tortillas	110	1 tortilla
Nature's Own	100% Whole Wheat Thin-Sliced Bagels	110	1 bagel

Brand	Whole-Grain Option	Calories	Serving Size
Pepperidge Farm	Very Thin 100% Whole Wheat Bread	110	3 slices
Pepperidge Farm	Farmhouse 100% Whole Wheat Bread	110	1 slice
Thomas'	100% Whole Wheat Bagel Thins	110	1 bagel thin
Thomas'	100% Whole Wheat Mini Bagels	110	1 mini bagel
Pepperidge Farm	100% Whole Wheat Hamburger Buns	120	1 bun
Thomas'	100% Whole Wheat English Muffins	120	1 muffin
Nature's Own	100% Whole Wheat English Muffins	120	1 muffin
Van's	Whole Grain Minis	120	8 minis
Arnold	Stone Ground 100% Whole Wheat Bread	130	2 slices
Oroweat	100% Whole Wheat Dinner Rolls	130	1 roll
Nature's Own	100% Whole Wheat Sandwich Rolls	130	1 roll
Thomas'	Thomas' Sahara 100% Whole Wheat Pita Pockets Mini Size	140	2 mini pitas*
Van's	Multi Grain Belgian Waffles	170	2 waffles
Van's	8 Whole Grains Waffles	170	2 waffles
Nature's Path	Ancient Grains Frozen Waffles	180	2 waffles

*Our plan uses 35-calorie mini pitas; substitute with half a Thomas' Sahara mini pita

Appendix

METRIC EQUIVALENTS

The recipes in this book use the standard United States method for measuring liquid and dry or solid ingredients (teaspoons, tablespoons, and cups). The information on these charts is provided to help cooks outside the U.S. successfully use these recipes. All equivalents are approximate.

METRIC EQUIVALENTS FOR DIFFERENT TYPES OF INGREDIENTS

A standard cup measure of a dry or solid ingredient will vary in weight depending on the type of ingredient. A standard cup of liquid is the same volume for any type of liquid. Use the following chart when converting standard cup measures to grams (weight) or milliliters (volume).

Standard Cup	Fine Powder (e.g., flour)	Grain (e.g., rice)	Granular (e.g., granulated sugar)	Liquid Solids (e.g., butter)	Liquid (e.g., milk)
1	140 g	150 g	190 g	200 g	240 ml
¾	105 g	113 g	143 g	150 g	180 ml
⅔	93 g	100 g	125 g	133 g	160 ml
½	70 g	75 g	95 g	100 g	120 ml
⅓	47 g	50 g	63 g	67 g	80 ml
¼	35 g	38 g	48 g	50 g	60 ml
⅛	18 g	19 g	24 g	25 g	30 ml

EQUIVALENTS FOR LIQUID INGREDIENTS BY VOLUME

¼ tsp. =				1 ml	
½ tsp. =				2 ml	
1 tsp. =				5 ml	
3 tsp. =	1 Tbsp. =		½ fl. oz. =	15 ml	
	2 Tbsp. =	⅛ cup =	1 fl. oz. =	30 ml	
	4 Tbsp. =	¼ cup =	2 fl. oz. =	60 ml	
	5⅓ Tbsp. =	⅓ cup =	3 fl. oz. =	80 ml	
	8 Tbsp. =	½ cup =	4 fl. oz. =	120 ml	
	10⅔ Tbsp. =	⅔ cup =	5 fl. oz. =	160 ml	
	12 Tbsp. =	¾ cup =	6 fl. oz. =	180 ml	
	16 Tbsp. =	1 cup =	8 fl. oz. =	240 ml	
	1 pt. =	2 cups =	16 fl. oz. =	480 ml	
	1 qt. =	4 cups =	32 fl. oz. =	960 ml	
			33 fl. oz. =	1000 ml	1 L

EQUIVALENTS FOR DRY INGREDIENTS BY WEIGHT

To convert ounces to grams, multiply the number of ounces by 30.

1 oz. =	¹⁄₁₆ lb. =	30 g
4 oz. =	¼ lb. =	120 g
8 oz. =	½ lb. =	240 g
12 oz. =	¾ lb. =	360 g
16 oz. =	1 lb. =	480 g

EQUIVALENTS FOR COOKING/OVEN TEMPERATURES

	Fahrenheit	Celsius	Gas Mark
Freeze Water	32°F	0°C	
Room Temperature	68°F	20°C	
Boil Water	212°F	100°C	
Bake	325°F	160°C	3
	350°F	180°C	4
	375°F	190°C	5
	400°F	200°C	6
	425°F	220°C	7
	450°F	230°C	8
Broil			Grill

EQUIVALENTS FOR LENGTH

(To convert inches to centimeters, multiply the number of inches by 2.5.)

1 in. =			2.5 cm	
6 in. =	½ ft =		15 cm	
12 in. =	1 ft =		30 cm	
36 in. =	3 ft =	1 yd =	90 cm	
40 in. =			100 cm =	1 m

DONATION ACKNOWLEDGMENTS

Good Housekeeping would like to thank the following companies, which generously contributed products to our 7 *Years Younger Anti-Aging Breakthrough Diet* panelists' starter kits:

Crest (3D Whitestrips): 3dwhite.com

Omron (pedometers): store.omronhealthcare.com

Dormtique (yoga mats): mycustomyogamat.com

Oxo (water bottles): oxo.com

Food Should Taste Good (Multigrain Chips): foodshouldtastegood.com

Kind Healthy Snacks (Mini Granola Bars): kindsnacks.com

The Vitamin Shoppe (omega-3 fish oil supplements): vitaminshoppe.com

Thomas' (Bagel Thins): thomasbreads.com

Van's Natural Foods (coupon for whole-grain waffles): vansfoods.com

Index

Week 6, 192
Week 7, 193
MET (metabolic equivalent), 153–155
Metric equivalents, 297–300
Mindset, 119–141
    adjusting, 82–83, 120–121
    de-nicing yourself, 133
    dieting styles and, 120–121
    importance of, 119–124
    letting go of emotional eating, 130, 132
    overview and activating *Diet* now,
        119–124, 141
    overworked, overwhelmed, overeating,
        137–138
    people-pleasing trap and, 131–133
    power of mind over stomach, 121–122
    setting goals, 95–96
    silencing mental saboteurs, 124–130. *See also*
        Cravings, controlling
    "thin," establishing, 138–140
    thrill-seeking and, 133–137
    visualization techniques, 139–140, 208, 211
    willpower and resolve, 113–116, 148
    writing reducing anxiety and, 128
Minerals. *See* Nutrients; *specific minerals*
Murray, Amy, 219
Muscle. *See also* Exercise
    building/firming, 40–41, 113, 134
    Diet and, 39–41
    losing, 39

N

Nebrow, Anne, M.D., 139
Nutrients. *See also* Carbohydrates; Fat; Fiber;
    Protein; *specific vitamins and minerals*
        in dairy, 41–43
        skin savers, 35–39
        supplements, 45

O

Obesity
    convenience foods and, 74–79
    Diet fighting, 28
    exercise and, 175
    fat/food intake and weight loss, 34
    trans fat and, 100
Oil vs. butter, 54
Omega-3 fatty acids, 43, 44, 45, 71–72, 184
Overworked, overwhelmed, overeating, 137–138

P

Panel, of successful losers
    about, 10–11
    advice and success tips from. *See specific*
        panelist names (listed on pages 5–6)

becoming panelist, 25
    names of, 5–6
    perspectives on *Diet* plan, 60–61
    perspectives on meal plan, 66–67
    recipes discussions, 218–219
    weight-loss successes, 11
Pantry, purging, 94
Patel, Alpa V., Ph.D., 145
Patrick, Maggie, 219
Pedometers, 152, 156, 208
People-pleasing, overcoming, 131–133
Permitters, 120–121
Pinterest.com, 25
Plateaus, 134, 165
Pledge, *Diet*, 19–23
    example, 20
    panelist pledges, 21–23
    preparing and posting, 89
    writing guidelines, 19–20, 89
Pork. *See Index of Recipes and Main Ingredients*
Portion control
    after seven weeks, 82
    checking/measuring portion sizes, 101, 102
    chips and, 194
    clean-plate club and, 101–102
    dining out and, 198–199, 202, 205
    dining ware size and, 103–104
    "family-style" dining and, 103
    frozen entrées and, 76
    gearing up for, 14–15, 28
    importance of, 183–184
    listening to your stomach, 104, 205
    panelist perspectives on, 31, 63, 81, 91, 101, 210
    weekend splurges and, 203
Poultry. *See Index of Recipes and*
    Main Ingredients
Prayer, 137
Prediabetes, 22
Protein
    animal/meats, 40, 68
    benefits and importance, 39–41, 67, 100
    calories from, 15, 40
    choosing, 40, 57
    in *Diet*, 64, 66, 67, 68
    muscle development and, 40–41
    nuts, 66
    proportion of meal, 64, 184
    skin health, wrinkles and, 41
    vegetarian, 188, 189
    weight loss and, 39–40
    what you'll eat, 41, 68
Purging pantry and fridge, 94

Q

Qi, Qibin, Ph.D., 157
Quercetin, 33, 38

INDEX OF RECIPES AND MAIN INGREDIENTS

Cover design by Jill Armus
Book design by Robert Campos

Photography Credits
Cover Image: © Depositphotos.com/konstantin32
Expert Team Photos: Photographs by PHILIP FRIEDMAN/Studio D
7YY Before Photos: Photographs by PHILIP FRIEDMAN/Studio D
7YY After Photos: Photographs by ALEX BEAUCHESNE
Exercise photos: Photographs by Jason Todd

Library of Congress Cataloging-in-Publication Data

7 years younger : the anti-aging breakthrough diet : lose 20 pounds (or more!) / by the editors of Good Housekeeping.
    pages cm
  Includes index.
  ISBN 978-1-936297-10-8 (hardcover : alk. paper) -- ISBN 1-936297-10-8 (hardcover : alk. paper) 1. Longevity--Nutritional aspects. 2. Aging--Prevention--Nutritional aspects. 3. Reducing diets--Recipes. I. Good housekeeping (New York, N.Y.) II. Title: Seven years younger.
  RA776.75.A12 2013
  613.2--dc23

                    2013023641

10 9 8 7 6 5 4 3 2 1

Published by Hearst Magazines
300 West 57th Street
New York, NY 10019

Good Housekeeping is a registered trademark and 7YY is a trademark of Hearst Communications, Inc.

www.goodhousekeeping.com

www.7yearsyounger.com

Distributed to the trade by Hachette Book Group

For information regarding discounts to corporations, organizations, non-book retailers and wholesalers; mail order catalogs; and premiums, contact:
Special Markets Department
Hachette Book Group
237 Park Avenue
New York, NY 10017
Call toll free: 1-800-222-6747
Fax toll free: 1-800-222-6902

All US and Canadian orders:
Hachette Book Group
Order Department
Three Center Plaza
Boston, MA 02108
Call toll free: 1-800-759-0190
Fax toll free: 1-800-286-9471

For all international orders:
Hachette Book Group
237 Park Avenue
New York, NY 10017
Tel: 212-364-1325
Fax: 800-364-0933
international@hbgusa.com

Printed in the USA